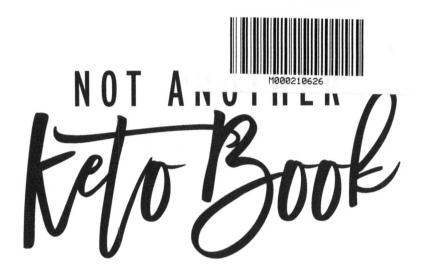

NOT ANOTHER Keto Book

The **Obesity Medicine Solution**
to Lose Weight, Boost Your
Metabolism, and Feel Great

Tuxedo Paw
PRESS

Contact information for Tuxedo Paw Press—tuxedopawpress@gmail.com

ISBN: 978-1-7369685-0-5 (print)
ISBN: 978-1-7369685-1-2 (ebook)

Ordering Information:
Special discounts are available on quantity purchases by corporations, associations, and others. For details, contact tuxedopawpress@gmail.com.

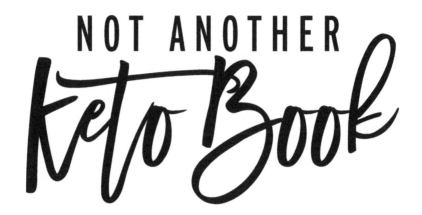

NOT ANOTHER Keto Book

The **Obesity Medicine Solution**
to Lose Weight, Boost Your
Metabolism, and Feel Great

Linda Anegawa, MD, MS, FACP, Dipl. ABOM

To my husband Ron, endless gratitude.

Your amazing cooking and incredible love

have nourished me all through the writing process.

DISCLAIMER

The aim of this book is to share my approach to obesity medicine and to discuss general concepts relating to metabolic health. It should not be taken as individual medical advice under any circumstances. Prior to beginning a weight-loss or diet program of any kind, you should always seek the advice of your personal physician.

TABLE OF CONTENTS

1

WHAT? ANOTHER WEIGHT-LOSS BOOK?

"I always consider that the shape of the future is in our hands. The past is past and can't be changed, but the future has not yet arrived."
—The Dalai Lama

Well, it's not exactly a "weight-loss book." This book is actually about Obesity Medicine. Let me explain the difference.

BACKGROUND

Over the last 50 years, Americans have gotten heavier and sicker, despite being advised to eat less and exercise more. Carrying excess weight goes hand-in-hand with poor metabolic health, and this condition has become one of the biggest threats to modern global health.[1] Metabolic syndrome repercussions include type 2 diabetes, hypertension, and cardiovascular disease, among many others.[2]

Metabolic health—as defined as having normal blood glucose, lipids, blood pressure, and body composition—has become more and more elusive, with data from the National Health and Nutrition Examination Survey in 2019 and the American Society of Clinical Endocrinologists showing that only 12% of Americans meet the definition of metabolic health.[3]

• FOOD for THOUGHT •
Markers of Good Metabolic Health[4] *

Fasting Glucose <100

Hemoglobin A1C <5.7%

Triglycerides <150

High-density lipoprotein (HDL) Cholesterol >40

Blood Pressure <130/85

Waist Circumference <35" if biologically female, <40" if biologically male

These numbers also assume that a person is not taking medications to control these factors (such as blood pressure or diabetes medications).

The higher our weight, the more likely we are to be metabolically unhealthy, particularly if excess weight is stored around the midsection. We know that belly weight behaves in an entirely different way hormonally than weight on the arms or legs and that it puts us at higher risk for cardiovascular disease and type 2 diabetes.[5]

In addition to the classic metabolic health parameters, our struggle with the COVID-19 pandemic has made it quite clear that metabolic health probably has a much broader definition to also include strong immunity and disease resistance. Data have been rapidly accumulated to indicate that metabolically unhealthy individuals are at the highest risk for severe disease and death from the coronavirus. Studies of over 40,000 COVID-19 patients treated at academic centers in New York City in March and April 2020 showed that a Body Mass Index (BMI) over 40 (roughly equivalent to being 100 lb. overweight) is one of the strongest predictors of hospitalization, even more so than being over the age of 65.[6]

Another study of over 6,000 patients within the Kaiser system showed that death rates from COVID-19 in younger patients were clearly linked to BMI.[7] This study was especially interesting given that other potential confounding factors that could increase death rates on their own, such as smoking, income disparity, and diseases like type 2 diabetes, were eliminated as possible influences.

COVID-19 and the aftermath has exploded like a bomb in our faces and shown us how our traditional approaches to disease care simply aren't working. Originating from the US Centers for Medicare and Medicaid Services, which declared in 2004 that "obesity is not a disease," an entire industry has sprung up with the premise that personal willpower is the key to weight loss.[8]

But we all know what happened: The "eat less, exercise more" mantra, billions of dollars in exercise programs, supplements, books, Instagram diet gurus or coaches, and quick fixes have all gotten us nowhere. In fact, we are in a far worse predicament than in 2004, when 32% of all Americans were classified as having morbid obesity: that number has mushroomed to over 42.4% per data released from the Centers for Disease Control and Prevention (CDC) in February 2020.[9]

WHAT IS OBESITY MEDICINE?

Okay, so back to this book and why I wrote it. In 2008, the Obesity Society—an organization of physicians, surgeons, and scientists dedicated to caring for patients with weight-related illness—gathered an expert scientific panel to review a rationale for labeling obesity as a disease for the very first time.[10] Historically, because of the relationship between one's weight and one's physical appearance, plus moral beliefs and weight-related discrimination, the superficial implications of excess weight have received far more attention than the medical ones.

Fortunately, the tide began turning in 2013 with the American Medical Association's recognition of obesity as a complex, chronic disease that requires medical attention.[11] This truly was a turning point over 30 years in the making! However, I find that most people are still reluctant to embrace obesity as a medical condition, and affected individuals continue to suffer from blame and embarrassment plus reduced access to the care that they so critically need.

As a double board-certified obesity medicine and internal medicine physician, I want readers to experience, as closely as possible, what a walk-through of my typical weight-management consultation visit looks like.

And while it's no secret that low-carbohydrate eating habits are a big part of my toolbox, I present a far more comprehensive *adapt and adjust* approach to overall life change, versus the more common weight-loss and maintenance approaches, which I feel only reinforce the black-and-white diet-mentality thinking that rarely leads to lasting change.

Notice that thinking about a plan to adapt and adjust is a very different mindset than most of us have when starting a new lifestyle program. We tend to think of ourselves as being either "on a diet" or "off a diet" (AKA cheating). Such a black-and-white approach to dieting has never led anyone to long-term success with health and wellness! That is why I vastly prefer the terms adapt and adjust: I believe they help to reinforce the concept that the changes we make are *not* a quick fix or something you are going to temporarily suck up so you can go back to eating junk food. That's not how metabolic health happens.

I will also address topics such as how to deeply explore *why* the journey is important to you, the basics of eating and lifestyle changes, and the use of adjunctive therapies such as medication and surgery to reinforce the process. We will troubleshoot together extensively in "Speedbumps and Roadblocks" (Chapter 8) with examples of real-life situations. And although I have included a chapter on maintenance—"Adapting and Adjusting for Life" (Chapter 11)—it's really just a continuation of the ongoing discussion.

I hope that my unique perspective, conveyed through this book, will be eye-opening compared to the mass-marketed, typical weight-loss advice. At the end of some chapters, when relevant, I also invite readers to complete self-exploration exercises to personalize information and to allow time to reflect on the concepts outlined.

The time has never been more critical for us to take excess weight seriously as a medical issue. We simply can't afford to ignore obesity, which took center stage as the elephant in the room of the COVID-19 crisis.[12] Even with our wonderful new vaccines, what about the next virus—COVID-21 or -22? We simply must fortify our metabolic health, as this is the only way to develop true disease resistance. Plus, *you* deserve a fresh, holistic, comprehensive approach combining the very best of what nutrition, lifestyle advice, and medical science has to offer.

Some final points to close out this chapter: in reading through this book, you'll hear me speak of a wide variety of approaches and techniques that can improve your metabolic health, from mindset shifts, to eating changes, to movement, medications, and even weight-loss surgery. While I will present this "buffet" of options for you to look over and savor, the decision on how to proceed is ultimately up to you. No two people, no two bodies, no two lives are ever alike. It's up to each of you as individuals to pick the approaches that speak most strongly to you and put together those puzzle pieces of how best to approach your health.

Please enjoy, and I hope to hear from you!

Linda Anegawa, MD, FACP

@metabolichealth4life_MD

2

DEFINE YOUR "WHY"

"To succeed, you need to find something to hold on to, something to motivate you, something to inspire you."
—*Tony Dorsett (ex-NFL star athlete)*[13]

It's the first thing I ask patients in my exam room after I introduce myself.

It's what I ask people to revisit again and again on their path, especially when motivation wanes.

It's what will keep you focused on your journey even when it seems like your hard work isn't paying off the way you want.

Before we begin the adapt and adjust process, it's critical to first ask yourself the following: *Why* do you want your weight to change? *Why* are you seeking help? *Why* now?

After you've adapted to a new way of eating, finding your *why* will help you make ongoing adjustments to your lifestyle to keep the progress going!

This will be your own personal *why* (or *why* list).

No one else's—it's different for everyone. And it's absolutely essential that you discover it for yourself.

What's the best way to figure out your unique *why*? Despite what you may think, it's not always an easy answer.

Try asking yourself the question now. You may hear yourself instinctively answering, "For better health," or "Because my doctor told me I need to," as top reasons.

But it's critical to get to the deeper *why*, as this is what you'll keep revisiting when life throws curveballs at you. And a shallow answer just won't suffice in keeping you engaged.

One way to find your *why* is to start asking yourself some more specific questions, such as:

1. **What bothers me about my weight?**

   There could be one reason, or there could be many. Perhaps you suffer from fatigue that you feel is weight related. You might be bothered by aches and pains. You might have mobility difficulties that limit you chasing your kids at the park. You might suffer from low self-esteem and wish for a better body image—in other words, to be more comfortable in your own skin. As one patient told me, "I feel like my body has become a prison, a trap, and I know I won't feel happy until I can get out." Another patient's words: "My body makes me feel like a failure." Powerful stuff.

2. **What do I hope to achieve with my weight loss? What are my goals?**

   A top reason I hear again and again is "To improve my health and get off my meds." Many of my patients were frightened by the COVID-19 situation and want to give themselves the best possible chance of resisting the impact of infection.

The best part is that you don't need to lose giant amounts of weight to do this. Extensive research shows that even a 5%–10% loss of weight can dramatically improve blood sugar, blood pressure, and cholesterol while also reducing joint pain.[14] In fact, often times the doses of medications taken for your chronic health conditions can be reduced even *before* weight is lost, simply because of low-carb eating changes. It's not necessarily all about the scale!

Other reasons can include: to live longer, to feel more at ease with yourself, to eventually feel more comfortable traveling (many of us have been dying to travel again), or even to attend a special event. One patient told me she wanted to set a weight-loss goal so she could dance at her son's upcoming wedding—something she couldn't do when we first met since her knees ached so much.

> ***Patient Voice:*** *MW (female, executive)*
>
> *"No matter what happens, I never want to go back to using my sleep apnea treatment machine again. That's the thought that keeps me focused through all the difficulties with changing my eating."*

3. **Who is the weight loss for?**

   Is it for your children, to set a good, healthy example for them? Is it to help improve your looks for those who might be viewing your profile on that dating app? Or is it finally something for *you*?

   Creating healthy lifestyle habits can definitely help to support a healthy weight once any underlying medical and/or hormonal influences are corrected. But these habits take time and energy. It's often too easy to justify not putting in the time—after all, most of us have families to care for, jobs, and other responsibilities. Putting our own bodies and health on the back-burner can, unfortunately, become habitual. A key component of defining your *why* may be a commitment to actually putting your own needs first for a change.

This third point may be the hardest for many of us. We all know we *should* be making healthy decisions and doing everything we can to put our own health first. But as so often happens, real life gets in the way.

There are family obligations, cranky kids, work struggles, unexpected curveballs and life crises (the pandemic sure was a big one), illnesses, financial difficulties, and a never-ending to-do list that always seem to gnaw at you.

HOW CAN WE GET AROUND THIS?

First, you *must* schedule "me time" regardless of what else is happening in your life. Put self-care on your calendar if you have to, so you are sure to do it! Even if it's something that seems really simple, like spending 30 minutes to veg alone on the couch with a great book, taking a hot bath, going for a quick walk, or enjoying a coffee with a friend. Time for yourself is critical for your resilience—by which I mean your ability to roll with the punches, reduce stress, and bounce back from difficulty. This may mean saying no to other things that are less critical, which is not easy for most of us. But practice it—it gets easier! And don't let excuses stand in your way.

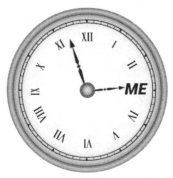

Schedule "Me Time"

Learning to delegate is also critical. Many of us want to feel we can handle it all ourselves, but the truth is we all need each other. Get your spouse or partner (or even your kids!) to help out more with chores around the house. At work, collaborate with others on big projects—working together will make everyone more efficient.

You may also want to think about setting just one small goal for yourself (not necessarily eating related) such as

- Drinking eight glasses of water daily,

- Resolving to take three deep breaths whenever you feel angry or stressed (I like to do this while sitting in the car in a traffic jam), or

- Taking the stairs instead of the elevator whenever possible. In this era of COVID-19 and its aftermath, it's good for social distancing, too!

After you achieve one small goal, try adding a second, or a third. Over time, you'll start feeling good about your accomplishments instead of feeling discouraged. This is a great place to start, even *before* you tackle the adapt and adjust process.

CHAPTER TAKEAWAY POINTS

The very first steps, prior to diving into the lifestyle change process are (1) defining your *why* and (2) identifying your weight-loss goals.

SELF-EXPLORATION

It's your turn! Think about what motivates you and write it down.

My Why(s):

_____

My Goal(s):

_____

How will I put myself first so I can achieve my goals?

_____

3

WHY LOW CARB?

"Four years of medical school, and four years of internship and residency, and I never thought anything was wrong with eating sweet rolls and doughnuts."
—Robert Atkins, MD

"We are now at a turning point in the history of ketogenic diets."
—Jeff Volek, PhD, RD and Stephen Phinney, MD, PhD[15]

"I'm going keto!"

Everywhere you turn, it seems that friends, family, and coworkers are talking about low-carbohydrate and ketogenic diets.

Celebrities swear by them.

Self-proclaimed social media influencers preach about their experiences of following them.

The medical establishment (mostly) raises their eyebrows at them.

Indeed, Google searches on the word "keto" outranked any other diet search in 2018 for the first time.[16] It was also in the top two trending health questions Googled in 2019, overtaking other top topics such as endometriosis, influenza, ALS, and "how long does weed stay in your urine."[17]

For the sake of simplicity, throughout this book I'll use the term "low carb" to include both ketogenic diets and low-carb diets.

• FOOD *for* THOUGHT •
Keto vs. Low Carb

While ketogenic diets are low in carbohydrates, not all low-carb diets are ketogenic. There are some important differences.

A ketogenic diet is a specific type of low-carb eating plan in which carbohydrates are kept very low, generally less than 20–30 g/day. This leads to a process called nutritional ketosis.[18] Ketosis is a process in which molecules called ketones are found in the bloodstream as a result of the breakdown of fat particles (called triglycerides) from fat cells.[19]

A low-carb diet reduces carbohydrates far lower than the US recommended daily dietary allowance of at least 225–300 g/day for a 2,000 calorie/day diet. Low-carb diets do not necessarily result in nutritional ketosis. Lowcarbusa.org defines varying degrees of low-carb eating, including moderate carbohydrate restriction (130+ g/day), reduced-carbohydrate diets (50–130 g/day), low-carbohydrate-ketogenic diets (30–50 g/day), and very low-carbohydrate/ketogenic diets (>30 g/day).[20]

What I love and appreciate about these guidelines is that they are highly customizable to individual patients—there is truly no "one size fits all." And although we may find it easy to adapt to one particular eating mode, being able to adjust later on to differing degrees of therapeutic carbohydrate restriction will be a critical part of ongoing lifestyle modifications that enable continued progress.

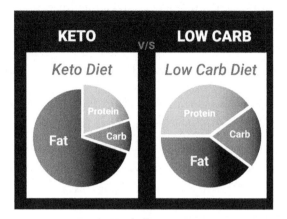

Keto Vs. Low Carb Nutrient Composition

WHERE DID LOW CARB COME FROM?

We often catch a few eye-rolls when low carb is mentioned, as in, "Are you really going to jump on the bandwagon of another fad diet?" But when you take a look at the history of this eating pattern, you really can't call it a fad at all.

In fact, the low-carb diet had its origin thousands of years ago when most of our ancestors lived a pretty carb-restricted lifestyle. Three hundred thousand years ago, most of the planet did not have access to a tropical environment where fruits were available throughout the year. Humans lived as mobile herders, following the animals that fed them. Europeans didn't have access to the potato until the sixteenth century, and agriculturally based carbohydrates such as wheat and rye only began to spread to northern Europe after the time of Christ. Therefore, many of our ancestors had very little exposure to dietary carbs until around just 1,500 years ago.[21] That's an incredibly brief time in human history!

Fast-forward to the modern history of carb restriction: many credit a British undertaker named William Banting for the founding of the modern-day low-carb diet. Banting had always struggled with his own weight no matter what he tried. He started by eating less and exercising more, but eventually his measures became increasingly extreme (including laxative use and near-starvation). However, he failed to get the results he wanted.

In 1862, a surgeon named Dr. William Harvey suggested that Banting try an eating program that was moderate in protein, high in fat, and banned sugars, sweets, and starches. Harvey's recommendations resulted in a 50-pound weight loss. Banting was so delighted with his results, he published a pamphlet, and the term "to bant" became known as meaning "to diet."[22]

• FOOD *for* THOUGHT •
Comparing High-Carb and Low-Carb Foods

Note that many foods which are considered "healthy" may contain high amounts of carbohydrates. This is only a brief list to give you a general idea.

HIGH CARB

Many fruits, especially tropical fruits like banana, mango, papaya

Pasta and noodles

Rice

Bread

Potatoes

Cookies

Crackers

Pretzels

Juices

Sugars (including natural sugars like honey and brown sugar)

Candy

LOW CARB

Meat (beef, chicken, pork)

Fish

Eggs

Tofu

Plain yogurt

Green leafy vegetables

Cruciferous vegetables (like broccoli, cauliflower)

Cheese

Cream

Flax seeds

Nuts

Some fruits (such as dark berries)

Oils (like coconut or olive oil)

Unsweetened coffee and tea

In the 1900s, low-carb diets were advocated by prominent physicians including Sir William Osler, Dr. Elliot P. Joslin, and Dr. Russell Wilder to treat not just excess weight but seizures and type 1 and type 2 diabetes, for which there were no available medical treatments at the time.[23] Low-carb eating was the standard of care, widely accepted and used for decades.

So how did low-carb diets fall out of favor? Some "credit" the growth of pharmaceutical companies, which developed and mass-marketed insulin and other drugs. These medications were certainly necessary, or in some cases, such as type 1 diabetes in particular, lifesaving. However, they likely also made it easier for people to be treated without having to change what they were eating.[24]

In addition, following President Eisenhower's heart attack in 1955, what came to be known as the diet–heart hypothesis was popularized by a professor at the University of Minnesota, Ancel Keys. Essentially, his hypothesis postulated that if you ate fat, your blood would be infiltrated by fat, leading to heart attacks.[25]

Despite a lack of good data, the advocates of this easy-to-grasp notion became very influential in selling it to the US government, which developed national dietary guidelines and, in 1992, the infamous food pyramid per the US Department of Agriculture in response.[26] So, low fat rather than low carb became a national standard, with dietary guidelines urging us to reduce our intake of saturated and total fat. And what happened to Americans since the 1950s under these guidelines? Unfortunately, it is evident that we became fatter and sicker, with obesity, diabetes, and metabolic disease rates skyrocketing out of control.[27]

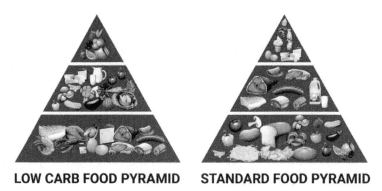

LOW CARB FOOD PYRAMID   STANDARD FOOD PYRAMID

Low-Carb Food Pyramid, Standard Food Pyramid

The tide of public opinion began to turn again in 1972 with the publication of *Diet Revolution* by Dr. Robert Atkins, a New York-based cardiologist.[28] The medical community was hostile; however, the book remained on the bestseller list for 285 weeks[29] and marked the start of once-dissenting voices chiming in, including the low-carb advocate Tim Noakes, a South

African scientist and ultramarathoner. Additionally, highly influential low-carb physician advocates such as Drs. Richard Bernstein, David Ludwig, and Mike Eades plus scientists such as Gary Taubes and Dave Feldman began contributing to the more balanced evaluation of low-carb eating.

Current data increasingly show that low-carb diets appear to be more effective than low-fat diets for the treatment of obesity and diabetes. In addition, a low-carb diet is felt to possibly carry other health benefits applicable to chronic inflammation, neurodegenerative conditions, and other diseases associated with insulin resistance.

Given that Americans have gotten heavier and sicker by following traditional dietary advice, it's easy to see how low-carb interventions have garnered a tremendous and growing amount of interest in the last five to six years. In caring for patients over the last two decades, I've personally never witnessed the degree of health improvements with my patients from *any* other intervention.

Without a doubt COVID-19 has exposed and further intensified the weaknesses in our traditional approaches to disease care and has led many to search for an alternate path to wellness—including *prevention*—which makes so much more sense. And when we speak of prevention, the traditional "eat less and exercise more" mantra really isn't cutting it, which is what mainly seems to be fueling the strong interest in low-carb eating—be it a classic ketogenic diet, vegetarian low carb, pescatarian keto, or whatever you like.

So, you are convinced that low carb is for you. Where do you even begin to get your information on how to proceed?

As soon as you start searching for keto diet plans, it quickly becomes apparent that everyone out there seems to be preaching the virtues of their own version. From Atkins to high fat to Mediterranean or even vegetarian preferences, you *can* eat low carb or keto with good results, as long as there is good eating consistency.

I believe this wholeheartedly; since not all obesity is the same problem, and no two bodies are alike, it's important to have a somewhat flexible and individualized approach.

There are many types of low-carb eating plans. The plan you choose should take into account not just your medical history and severity of metabolic disease but also your personal preference and lifestyle if you are to maintain and sustain your new eating plan and keep things consistent. Otherwise, you'll find yourself "on a diet" that you can't stick to, which will then, of course, lead you to going "off the diet" and making your body even sicker than when you started.

You've tried umpteen different things to address your weight, and you're ready for something different. Or maybe your weight is less of a concern, and you are more interested in some of the other reported health benefits of cutting carbs.

• FOOD *for* THOUGHT •
Potential Health Benefits of Lowering Carbohydrate Intake:[30]

Improved immune defenses (critical for thriving in the post-COVID-19 era)

Reduced weight

Improved blood sugar control

Diabetes remission

Cholesterol improvement

Blood pressure improvement

Fatty liver improvement

Better mood

Better energy

Less bloating

Whatever your reason, the low-carb craze has piqued your curiosity enough, and you are ready to go, guns blazing. But before you dive in, let's have a closer look at what low carb means for the body.

Science notwithstanding, as I stated earlier, I firmly believe that there is no one-size-fits-all approach.

But here's what low-carb approaches *do* have in common: they aim to activate the body's own natural fat-burning machinery. Becoming "fat-adapted" in this way taps into the excellent fueling system that we already have in our bodies, keeping our energy levels more even than if we relied primarily on dietary starch for energy.[31]

When we are fat-adapted, we can also achieve very efficient, and safe, weight loss. I think this is a critical point since lifestyle change can feel like a challenge. Why make the process even more challenging by fighting against the body? We have enough hurdles to contend with every day: preparing to go to work while getting kids ready for school, fighting traffic, dealing with common life stresses, etc.

Another hurdle that my patients commonly face is their high weight "set point." What do I mean by this? Well, we are learning that when weight is gained, the body then will see the new higher weight as normal, and it will fight against your efforts to dip below this.[32]

While it sounds incredibly unfair, it does makes sense from a biological standpoint. After all, as human animals, our three main evolutionary imperatives are (1) to reproduce, (2) to sleep, and (3) to eat—which of course helps us to accomplish (1) and (2). Most of us have bodies that hoard fat *very* efficiently, as this trait likely helped us to survive as cave people millions of years ago. Unfortunately, in the present day, our fat-hoarding biological tendencies work against us given that it is far easier to obtain our food sources: now, we can go to the drive-thru to satisfy hunger, rather than spending days or even weeks hunting a herd of antelope.

THE SCIENCE OF LOW-CARB EATING

First, what is a carbohydrate?

All carbohydrates are strings of sugar molecules bonded together. When we eat carbs, the body breaks them down into sugar molecules during the process of digestion. Therefore, eating any carbs—no matter how "healthy" they are—will increase blood sugar.[33]

Image of Carbohydrate Molecule + Sugar Molecule Components

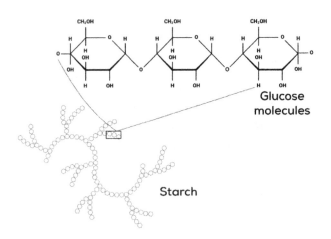

Despite what many people believe, it's interesting to note that carbohydrates are not considered to be essential nutrients for human life. The only nutrients we actually need to survive are proteins, fats, and micronutrients like certain vitamins and minerals.[34]

However, even though we don't need carbohydrates to survive, we do need sugar in our blood.[35] Tiny amounts are necessary for proper function of the organs and brain. Normally, our bodies have less than one teaspoon of sugar in the blood. This exquisitely controlled blood sugar level is regulated largely by a hormone called insulin.

Insulin is a hormone made by the pancreas, an organ in the belly right behind the stomach. Insulin's job is to drive blood sugar into our cells after a meal so that the amount of sugar in the blood doesn't get too high.

Insulin generally does a fantastic job at this and keeps blood sugar amounts incredibly tightly controlled in that one teaspoon range. Its mission to lower sugar is critical: once blood sugar becomes abnormally elevated, all sorts of health problems can arise. Chronically elevated blood sugar is indeed *toxic* to our bodies.[36]

• FOOD *for* THOUGHT •
Insulin and Glucagon

Insulin's partner hormone in blood sugar control is called glucagon, and they operate in opposite ways, almost like a seesaw.

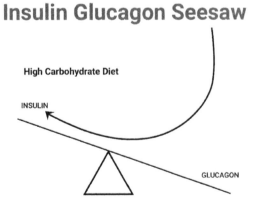

Insulin Glucagon Seesaw

High Carbohydrate Diet

INSULIN

GLUCAGON

Insulin mainly helps to lower blood sugar, while glucagon helps to raise it if it gets too low by directing the liver to produce more glucose in a process called gluconeogenesis.[37] Because of this, we don't need to eat carbohydrates to survive—our liver is perfectly capable of producing all the glucose we need.

In susceptible people the insulin control system can, unfortunately, break down over time. When blood sugar is chronically high, the body releases more insulin to try to compensate. But, unfortunately, this doesn't help, because over time the body becomes less and less effective at responding to insulin so that insulin, in turn, has a harder time pushing blood sugar out of the bloodstream into the body's cells and therefore lowering blood sugar. People who are susceptible to the body's insulin system breaking down are said to have metabolic syndrome, otherwise known as insulin resistance, or carbohydrate intolerance.

The result of the failure to respond to insulin is that blood sugar slowly rises over time and may even become dangerously high. It actually doesn't take much of a rise in blood sugar to cause diabetes—when sugar gets any greater than 1.25 tsp in the blood you've got yourself that dreaded diagnosis.

• FOOD *for* THOUGHT •

Symptoms or Signs That You Could Be Affected with Metabolic Syndrome[38]

History of difficulty losing weight or weight loss followed by regain

Strong family history of diabetes or prediabetes

Elevated blood pressure or cholesterol

History of gestational diabetes or abnormal glucose of any kind

Irregular menstrual periods (if you are biologically female)

Darkening of the skin around the neck (known as acanthosis nigricans)

With insulin resistance or carbohydrate intolerance, not only does sugar build up in the blood but insulin does as well. And high insulin turns out to be just as much of a problem as high blood sugar. The reason for this is that besides helping to regulate blood sugar, insulin is also one of our key fat-storage hormones.[39] The more sugar we add to a broken sugar-control system, the more insulin we will need and the less sensitive we become to insulin over time.

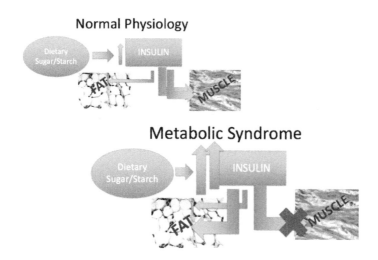

High insulin levels also cause other physiological disruptions, such as wrecking hormonal control of the menstrual cycle resulting in infertility,[40] increased inflammation leading to joint disorders,[41] and increased fat accumulation in the liver leading to non-alcoholic liver disease, which affects around 100 million Americans and has doubled in the past 20 years.[42]

Hyperinsulinemia, the condition that results from the body's broken sugar-control system can also be produced another way—by us doctors! When insulin is prescribed to lower a patient's blood sugar, this extra insulin in the body has the exact same effect as the extra insulin that we overproduce. If you have diabetes, you may have noticed weight gain and increased hunger when starting insulin shots. This is the reason why.

• FOOD *for* THOUGHT •
But Can't I Eat Some Carbs? Aren't Some Carbs Healthy?

Short answer: Yes, and yes. In fact, it is not possible to avoid all carbohydrates as there are small amounts even in low-carb foods like meats and green vegetables.

But it's important to understand that you may become ill from eating even just slightly too many carbs. Just like some people are lactose intolerant, you can be carb intolerant too, as we discussed above.

Carb intolerance can be a matter of degrees. We all have our personal threshold of how much carbohydrate we can eat before blood sugar starts rising—in other words, everyone has their own unique carb-tolerance level. Some people can eat carbs all day long and be perfectly fine, but others will develop metabolic syndrome and, eventually, even type 2 diabetes.

Here's an analogy, even though the physiology is different. Consider how much alcohol you can drink before you become intoxicated. I can have no more than 230 ml (around eight ounces) of wine; you may be able to drink more, or perhaps you can have none at all. How much your blood sugar spikes after carb ingestion is just as individual.

Now that you understand how the physiology of the blood glucose control system works, it becomes clear as to how continuing to eat over your personal carb-tolerance level can start you on a dangerous cycle. If you have metabolic syndrome, a carbohydrate-based diet is guaranteed to keep insulin levels high, which will keep the body trapped in fat-storage mode.

But by eating low carb (below your carb-tolerance level), insulin release decreases. Less insulin released means less fat storage, plus you unlock the body's natural ability to use stored fat as energy. The roots of metabolic disease are treated, insulin resistance goes down, and your health improves. And the other beautiful thing?

If carbs are low enough for this hormonal engine to work, then no calorie counting or exercise is generally needed to reverse the cycle and begin losing weight!

Why is this? This picture explains things more simply.

How Low Carb Works

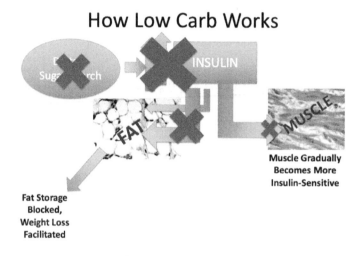

Muscle Gradually Becomes More Insulin-Sensitive

Fat Storage Blocked, Weight Loss Facilitated

Don't get me wrong: daily movement is healthy for our cardiovascular system, critical for regulation of mood, stress, and sleep, and helps boost our motivation. But it usually will not result in weight loss on its own. We'll delve further into this subject in Chapter 9, but please take my word on it for now.

The overall goal of low-carb eating, then, is to achieve optimal metabolic health, as defined previously, as easily as possible.

CHAPTER TAKEAWAY POINTS

Low-carb eating plans are *not* fad diets and can be a safe, healthy, and time-honored approach to weight loss.

A low-carb approach can take advantage of your body's innate fat-burning machinery to help you.

Low-carb diets can be individualized to meet almost anyone's needs and preferences, from carnivore to plant-based and everything in between.

Now that you know how it works, let's prepare to start!

SELF-EXPLORATION

What appeals to me about considering a low-carb lifestyle to improve my health?

_____

What potential obstacles exist for me?

_____

4

PREPARING TO START

"What lies behind you and what lies in front of you, pales in comparison to what lies within you."
—Albert Jay Nock

In preparing to start your journey to adapt and adjust to low-carb eating habits for weight loss, there are four critical items to address:

Your *goals*

Your *motivation* and *readiness* to adapt to change

Optimizing your medical conditions

Let's break things down one by one.

YOUR GOALS

Goal setting is a critical part of how you will adapt to lifestyle change. How do you know where you'll finish if you don't have something to aim for?

Having said that, our goals need to be doable and realistic. There is no such thing as a "miracle" diet, pill, or even surgery.

In addition, genetics plays a large role in our body shape.[43] If you come from a family where everyone is six feet tall and rail thin, there's a good chance you'll have this type of body. If your family is more solidly built, pear shaped, apple shaped, etc., your body will generally retain these characteristics, no matter your weight. And that's okay!

Because of this, I don't believe in the concept of an "ideal weight." Many of us have looked up this number and found online algorithms that tell you to start at 100 lbs. and add 5 lbs. per inch over five feet of height to arrive at the "ideal body weight" or something silly like this. It really is total nonsense. This formula was invented by life insurance companies to justify charging us higher premiums, and the calculation is not at all based on fact.

WHAT ABOUT BODY MASS INDEX (BMI)?

The BMI is a calculation based on weight and height only. These charts identify an "ideal" BMI as between 18.5 and 24.9—above this range, and you are classified as overweight. For example, if you are five feet, six inches tall, a BMI in this range would mean you should weigh between 118 and 155 lbs.[44]

However, what most people do not know is that the BMI was intended to be used as a research tool only, and not for widespread clinical practice as it is used today. The BMI also tells you nothing about body composition (body fat), which can make a huge difference.[45]

For example, it's entirely possible for a six-foot, four-inch-tall NFL linebacker with 10% body fat to have exactly the same BMI as a five-foot, two-inch sedentary accountant with 45% body fat!

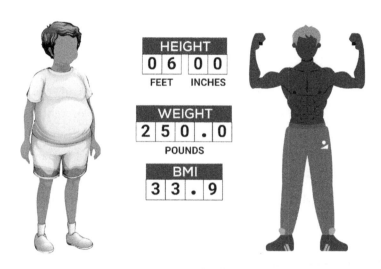

In this case, BMI does nothing to identify which one of these individuals is at risk from excess weight.

Here's something else to consider: regardless of whether there truly is an "ideal body weight," and if so how we should define it, there is also substantial research that shows that a modest weight loss of even 5%–10% can dramatically improve weight-related conditions, improve blood testing (such as blood sugar, cholesterol, and kidney numbers), and allow medications to be reduced or eliminated.[46] Not to mention how much better it can make you feel!

Therefore, I believe no one, not even your doctor, can tell you exactly what you "should" weigh. For every individual there is likely a wide range of weights within which our bodies can be healthy.

This is why I advise my patients not to fixate on a magic number. For example, you might even set a weight-loss goal of five pounds at a time and see how you and your body feels. A five-pound weight loss is often enough to really start to see a difference. Your final target weight might be something that we approach gradually as a process of discovery. After you adapt to a new way of eating, your goals are something that we can and should adjust over time.

And finally: the way I encourage patients to define their success is *far* more than just a number on the scale. There are so many other important ways to measure lifestyle change success: feeling better or lighter, experiencing less pain, reducing medications, getting off a sleep apnea machine, improved blood tests, fitting into clothes better, elevated self-image, and improved mood. You may not hit your high-school weight, but if you can come off your diabetes medication and have more energy to chase your kids around the house, I'd sure call that success, wouldn't you?

YOUR MOTIVATION AND READINESS TO ADAPT TO CHANGE

I often ask my patients, "How motivated are you?" and "How ready are you?" These may seem somewhat similar questions, but although they are related, they are really two different concepts. Let me clarify:

Motivation = drive and desire to get things done

Readiness = willingness and ability to put together and carry out a plan

For example, you might have all the motivation in the world. You might be sick and tired of feeling sick and tired. You might be yearning to fit back into those favorite jeans. Adapting to a healthier "you" may be something you have dreamed about for years.

But despite feeling motivated, you may not feel ready. The COVID-19 pandemic has forced many of us to adapt to a "new normal," and may have drained your energy down to an all-time low point. You might feel confused about what is the best path to take to achieve your goals. You might also feel overwhelmed about all of life's stressors and responsibilities including work, kids, running a home, and finances.

The idea of trying to adjust your lifestyle, after adjusting to so much during the pandemic, may even be terrifying for some. You might have tried and failed so many times before that you have a sense of helplessness about the process, or "diet fatigue." All these things can sap your readiness (and eventually they can harm your motivation, as well).

> **Patient Voice:** BV *(female, case worker)*
>
> *"I can't wait to be skinny, skinny, skinny! But my life is so crazy and that gets me down."*

Here are some suggestions to help you get *ready* and stay *motivated* for this process:

— Set realistic goals (per above).

— Give yourself small windows of time to prepare. Calendar the dates and times that you'll devote to shopping and meal prepping. If you are used to eating a lot of takeout and fast food, one hour twice a week is a great start for most people and should be easy to commit to. Remember: the more you prepare, the less likely it is you'll get off track.

— Clean out your pantry and your fridge. Your willpower is a finite resource! If you have to count on willpower every time you open the cupboard and see junk food, it will be much, much more difficult for you to succeed. Have a frank discussion with the people you live with and make sure to tell them what *you* need in order to be consistent with good eating habits. And throw away all the junk food or come up with an alternate arrangement—one patient of mine even purchased his own fridge to keep in his garage, which helped him to see the upstairs communal fridge contents as "off limits" for him.

— Block off 10 minutes each day to be alone with your thoughts and feelings. You could take a brief walk, meditate, or even turn the phone off and treat yourself to an uninterrupted hot shower.

33

- Reach out to others for support. The more you involve friends, family members, or coworkers, the better chance you'll have of succeeding.

- Start planning your rewards now! Not in the form of cupcakes or ice cream, but nonfood-related, meaningful rewards such as buying the new dress you've been eyeing or treating yourself to a pedicure.

On the other hand, if you find yourself not quite motivated yet to begin adapting to a new lifestyle, that's also worthwhile to note. Motivation naturally waxes and wanes depending on what else is going on in your life.

If you truly feel unmotivated, it might be worth taking a step back for a month and revisiting your goals at a later time. If you try to force yourself for whatever reason, when you are really not feeling it, how likely do you think you'll be to succeed? Don't beat yourself up or keep banging your head against the wall. Give yourself a little time to reflect.

In summary, remember:

1. There is no "ideal body weight"—the concept of the ideal body *range* is a lot more accurate.

    Your *function* is more important than the scale.

    Your *medical* goals are more important than the scale.

    How you *feel* is more important than the scale!

2. Motivation and readiness are two separate concepts. Your plan to be *ready* to adapt to changes should be designed to back up how *motivated* you are to be on the journey at the outset.

A WORD FOR WOMEN OF CHILDBEARING AGE

If you are of childbearing age, planning a pregnancy, or are currently pregnant, the discussion on readiness for you will have particular relevance. It is estimated that approximately 25% of women who are currently pregnant suffer from obesity and as such are at high risk from obesity-related poor pregnancy outcomes, including gestational diabetes and hypertensive disorders of pregnancy.[47] These conditions put both mother and baby's health at substantial risk during pregnancy as well as after childbirth. Data suggests that weight loss pre-pregnancy, or even during pregnancy, can reduce the rate of adverse pregnancy outcomes. However, I passionately believe that anyone who is currently pregnant or contemplating a pregnancy should work closely with their physician to make sure that any weight-loss program is done in a safe and healthful manner.

OPTIMIZING YOUR MEDICAL CONDITIONS

Prior to starting work with a new patient, I like to make sure medical conditions in the body are as finely tuned as they can be to adapt to the weight-loss process. What do I mean by this?

One example is eliminating medical obstacles to weight loss. Do you know that there is an enormous number of medications that can block weight loss or make it more difficult? Here is a partial list of known offenders, but there are plenty of other medications that can also affect body weight.

Diabetes medications[48]

- Insulins

- Sulfonylureas (examples: glyburide, glipizide, glimepiride, tolazamide)

- Thiazolidinediones (rosiglitazone, pioglitazone)

- Meglitinides (repaglinide, nateglinide)

Cardiovascular medications[49]

- Beta-blockers (propranolol, atenolol, metoprolol)

- Older calcium channel blockers (nifedipine, amlodipine, felodipine)

35

Antidepressants and other psychoactive drugs[50]

- Tricyclics (amitriptyline, doxepin, imipramine)

- *Some* serotonin enhancers (paroxetine, citalopram, sertraline, duloxetine)

- Others: phenelzine, isocarboxazid, mirtazapine, brexpiprazole, desvenlafaxine, olanzapine, quetiapine, clozapine, risperidone, zotepine

Hormones or hormone modulators[51]

- Glucocorticoid hormones (steroids)

- Tamoxifen

- Aromatase inhibitors

- Estrogens and progestins (common birth control ingredients)

Seizure or pain medications[52]

- Carbamazepine, gabapentin, valproate, pregabalin, divalproex, lithium, cariprazine

Miscellaneous[53]

- Diphenhydramine (Benadryl), some HIV medications, cyclophosphamide, 5-fluorouracil

If you are on any of these medications, please talk to your doctor. A gradual dose reduction or substitution may be a big help. *But* a word of caution: **do *not* stop any medications on your own!** Doing so can be extremely dangerous if not supervised by a physician.

There are other conditions that I look for as well that can interfere with our ability to adapt and adjust to the weight-loss process. For example, hormone issues such as adrenal or thyroid conditions, sleep apnea, abnormally low muscle mass, heart failure, certain types of tumors (pituitary tumors or an insulinoma), chronic stress or depression, or even a rare genetic disorder causing obesity are all conditions I screen for carefully when I meet new patients.

CHAPTER TAKEAWAY POINTS

Readiness to start a lifestyle change program, beyond goal setting, involves a clear and realistic assessment of your motivation and readiness. It's also critical to work with your physician to optimize your health so that any conditions you may have don't stand in your way!

Motivated *and* ready to get started?

SELF-EXPLORATION

1. *My goals*:

   _____

2. *My motivation level* to adapt to changes (circle):

   High   Medium-High   Medium   Medium-Low   Low

   a. What are the key factors in my life that increase my motivation?

   b. What factors decrease my motivation?

3. *My readiness level* to adapt to changes (circle):

   High   Medium-High   Medium   Medium-Low   Low

   a. What factors increase or decrease my readiness?

4. My medical conditions to discuss with my physician prior to beginning to adapt and adjust:

   _____

5

ADAPTING TO FUELING

"One Day, or Day One."
—Unknown

"I can. I will. End of story."
—Unknown

Now for the fun part—here we go!

This chapter will be somewhat interactive, so I'd encourage you to take notes where indicated to start to customize your own plan.

Keep in mind from earlier chapters the importance of your *why* and of being realistic about your goals.

- The vast majority of people on their quest for better health are not meant to look like scrawny fashion models or perfectly buff ironmen/women with less than 10% body fat. Genetics shape our shapes. Spend some time looking at family photos. If your parents, cousins, and grandparents are all pear shaped, it is unlikely that you'll be able to achieve a goal of having stick-figure-skinny legs, no matter how much weight you lose.

— Metabolic health can cover far more than what your glucose and lipids show. Strong immunity, disease resistance, absence of inflammatory symptoms or chronic pain, mental and emotional clarity, and a positive body image all play a role in optimal health, too!

— There is no "ideal body weight"—rather, for every individual there is a broad range of weights at which our bodies can be healthy.

— Success is far more than a number on the scale. Remember the other important measures of lifestyle change success: feeling better or lighter, reduced pain, reduced medication, improved blood test results, clothes fitting better, having more energy, enjoying a more positive outlook, etc. We may be aiming for a variety of results when we look to measure success.

Last, but not least: it's more important to listen to your body's signals rather than trying to count calories. Avoid rigidity over portion sizes and macros.

In approaching fueling, remember that this is a two-phase process: we adapt, and then we adjust to keep our progress moving forward.

Adapting is your initial active change process—it is designed for quicker results and changes.

Adjusting is your fine-tuning and tweaking as we go along—it is designed more for ongoing scale movement and to prepare you for optimum health maintenance.

In general, you should expect the adapt process of a lifestyle change to take approximately two to four weeks, though this varies by the individual and depends on many factors, including how many changes you incorporate.

For some people, adapting is relatively easy. Perhaps you are someone who has a supportive spouse to help with all your meal prepping and cooking to keep you on track; perhaps you have a relatively easy job (or you may even be retired!) and, therefore, can afford the time to dedicate to your new plan. If that is the case, you should be able to quickly and easily adapt to change by the two-week mark.

If, however, you are someone who has a more complex lifestyle (working multiple jobs, less schedule flexibility, a large family, or little support), adapting may take up to a month and would be better accomplished in a series of small changes that gradually build up.

There is no right or wrong approach; the adapting process will be different depending on who you are and your life circumstances.

In the fueling process, switching between the adapt and adjust phases is fluid. At any one given time, you may be solidly within a phase or combining both phase features. Your goals and your overall health profile define how long you are likely to spend in the adapt and adjust phases.

Within the adapt and adjust phases, there are both fueling (eating) and flowing (lifestyle balance) goals.

Phase 1: Adapt	*Fueling *Flowing
Phase 2: Adjust	*Fueling *Flowing

STARTING TO ADAPT THROUGH FUELING

Think: *Fuel up to power through* your entire day.

Principle: What we eat powers our body to do all the miraculous things it does every day.

Fuel pumps our heartbeat, ignites our nervous system, and enriches our circulation with energy, vitamins, and minerals.

Proper fueling allows us to withstand the tough times as well as the more minor day-to-day pressures and stress that add up over time. It also ensures that the body will find its way to its optimal individual weight.

BASE FUEL: "PROTEINS AND GREENS"— ESSENTIAL NUTRIENTS FOR THE BODY EVERY DAY

Every meal you eat should be based first and foremost on protein. Whether you eat one meal a day or four, a protein base is critical. Protein, and its building blocks, called amino acids, together form all bodily structures. Protein is an essential macronutrient because our bodies can't produce amino acids on their own—therefore we must take in protein in our food. You can eat plant-based or animal-based protein, however animal protein has higher biological value. This means that animal protein can be more easily converted to body protein.[54]

How much protein you should aim for is somewhat controversial and depends on a variety of factors including how active you are and how much you carb restrict.

The US recommended daily allowance calculator for protein intake is commonly cited by many dietary and fitness professionals.[55] It recommends 0.8 g per 1 kg (roughly two pounds) of body weight. For a 200-lb. individual, this would equal approximately 72 g of protein daily. However, this may underestimate the protein needs of many; particularly when on a low-carb eating plan, extra protein may be necessary.[56] Other studies have cited weight loss and lean mass preservation benefits with eating 20–30 g of protein per meal—this is critical, since when we are losing weight, we want to lose fat mass, not lean (muscle, bone, and nerve) mass.[57]

Overall, rather than doing complex calculations, I'd vastly prefer for you to listen to your body's hunger and satiety signals. But in the beginning, it's not a bad idea to use the above guidelines to give you a general idea of where you should be headed with protein consumption. Anywhere from 0.8–2 g/kg of body weight is likely safe and healthy; even if you eat more protein than the US RDA recommends, you'll still be falling within their recommended guidelines that state that calories from protein should be between 10%–35% of your total daily intake.

For your protein choices, you can use any preparation you wish including stir-frying, broiling, grilling, or simmering, as long as breading or sweet sauces are avoided. In addition, there is no need to remove fat from the protein that you eat.

SAMPLE LIST OF PROTEINS

- Fish including sashimi, lomilomi salmon, and poke (if made with sugar-free sauce)
- Shellfish (shrimp, prawns, scallops, clams, mussels, oysters)
- Beef
- Pork
- Chicken or poultry
- Tofu or tempeh or other vegetarian protein options (Beyond Meat, Impossible Burger, Morningstar Farms® products, Tofu Pups, etc.)
- Edamame—also contains carbohydrates
- Eggs and egg products
- Full-Fat dairy: cream, whole milk, Greek yogurt—also contains fat
- All cheeses—also contains fat

- Protein products like jerky (beef, turkey, fish)—look for the lowest-carb brand you can find.

- Deli meats—look for unprocessed or natural as much as possible.

- Protein bars—look for brands containing five grams or less net carbs such as Adapt Your Life, Ketobars, Premier Protein, Atkins, and Kirkland Signature Gluten-Free Protein bar brands.

- Protein shakes—look for brands containing three grams or less net carbs such as Premier Protein, Vega Protein & Greens, Muscle Milk 100% Whey, and Atkins.

GREENS

Green vegetables are important. They provide critical micronutrients (vitamins and minerals) for muscle and nerve function. Two to four cups daily (measured raw) are generally sufficient to provide adequate micronutrients. In choosing your vegetables, try to pick leafy and green choices as much as possible, as they are richest in fiber and micronutrient content.

SAMPLE LIST OF GREENS

Spinach	Kimchi	Wakame
Kale	Limu	Bamboo shoots
Salad greens—any kind	Mung bean sprouts	Broccoli
Chinese cabbage	Taro leaf	Brussel sprouts
Cucumber	Celery	Asparagus
Bok choy	Leaf lettuces	Peppers
Choy sum	Nori or dried seaweed	Green beans
Collard greens	Artichokes	Arugula

What about other veggies? Here are some examples and how they fit in:

Tomatoes—actually a fruit, but they are low in carbohydrates and provide flavor and micronutrients. Small amounts are fine.

Onions—although, be aware that cooking the onions releases large amounts of sugars. Does that sound a little nitpicky, especially since earlier I suggested you try not to be overly concerned with amounts and portions? Perhaps it does, however, remember that carbohydrates from multiple sources can quickly add up.

Cauliflower—similar in content to broccoli but just not green. Feel free to include.

Eggplant—somewhat higher in starch, but fine to use one-half cup, cooked, daily.

Starchy veggies (corn, carrots, potatoes)—see below under "Extras."

FATS

The fat we eat provides what are known as essential fatty acids, which give energy to the body and are a major component of our cells' membranes. Dietary fat also allows our bodies to absorb enough of the fat-soluble vitamins such as vitamins A, E, D, and K.

Eat natural fats to the point of satiety. The right amount of healthy fats will minimize cravings and help you to feel satisfied, *not* deprived. In addition, although saturated fats have been demonized, they have not been conclusively shown to contribute to adverse outcomes of any kind.[58] Listen to your body's signals. Aim for monounsaturated or saturated fats and avoid processed or polyunsaturated fats (like seed oils and margarine) as well as trans fats (partially hydrogenated fats).

SAMPLE LIST OF FATS

- Butter
- Olive oil
- Canola oil (for high-heat cooking)

- Coconut oil
- MCT oil
- Avocado
- Flax seed, chia seed, hemp hearts (especially if you are vegan)
- One-fourth cup of nuts or seeds (not trail mix) or two tablespoons unsweetened nut butter. Note that I'm giving portion sizes here because these items contain significant amounts of carbohydrate as well as fats and protein.
- Olives
- Cheeses (also a protein source)
- Fatty fish (like salmon)

Seasonings—basically, anything is okay if it's sugar-free.

- Fresh or dried herbs and spices
- Bonito flakes
- Hawaiian sea salt or Himalayan salt
- Miso paste—note that this has four grams of carbohydrate per tablespoon.
- Sugar-free dressings—olive oil or cream-based are the best. Also, Walden Farms brand is okay.
- Sugar-free sauces—like tomato sauce or curry paste but watch ingredients for any hidden carbs.

EXTRAS—NONESSENTIAL NUTRIENTS (OPTIONAL)

Although the body does not require these foods, if desired, one to two servings per day can help provide variety and flexibility to your eating and is reasonable for many people to try when they start. Keep in mind that adjustments to these amounts may be needed if the starter portion of one to two servings per day puts you over your individual carb threshold.

Some of these extras contain sugars, such as the fruits and some of the higher-starch veggies (peas, for example). Because the amounts they contain are relatively small and because they have other health benefits, these foods are permitted in small amounts. Do watch out for the many names for sugar in ingredients tables—it can be *very* misleading. Over 68% of barcoded food products contain added sugar in one form or another.[59]

• FOOD *for* THOUGHT •
What's in a Name?

Sugar by *all* these names is still sugar!

Anna Barwell listed 56 different names for sugar in an article on Virta Health's website, including:[60]

1. Dextrose	10. Cane juice crystals	19. Brown rice syrup
2. Fructose	11. Cane sugar	20. Buttered sugar or buttercream
3. Galactose	12. Caster sugar	21. Caramel
4. Glucose	13. Coconut sugar	22. Carob syrup
5. Lactose	14. Corn syrup solids	23. Corn syrup
6. Maltose	15. Crystalline fructose	24. Evaporated cane juice
7. Sucrose	16. Agave nectar or syrup	25. Yellow sugar
8. Beet sugar	17. Barley malt	26. Turbinado sugar
9. Brown sugar	18. Blackstrap molasses	27. Sucanat
28. Date sugar	38. Panela sugar	48. Fruit juice concentrate
29. Fruit juice	39. Demerara sugar	49. Maple syrup
30. Dextrin	40. Invert sugar	50. Golden syrup
31. Malt syrup	41. Diastatic malt	51. High-Fructose corn syrup (HFCS)
32. Molasses	42. Ethyl maltol	52. Maltodextrin

33.	Raw sugar	43.	Florida crystals	53.	Rice syrup
34.	Icing sugar	44.	Golden sugar	54.	Refiner's syrup
35.	Honey	45.	Glucose syrup solids	55.	Sorghum syrup
36.	Rice syrup	46.	Grape sugar	56.	Muscovado sugar
37.	Treacle	47.	Sugar (granulated or table)	57.	Confectioner's sugar (powdered sugar)

Notice here that in this extras section I am going to start to add in and discuss portions and measuring sizes. Why? Remember that if you have metabolic syndrome, your body does not process carbohydrates effectively or efficiently. If eaten in excess, these carbohydrates can increase insulin levels and then be stored, unfortunately, as fat, so we do need to account for them.

Fruits and vegetables

- Dark berries (blueberries, strawberries, raspberries), one-half cup/day

- Apple, one-half medium/day

- Dried unsweetened coconut, 2 tbsp/day

- Starchy veggies or tubers (carrot, sweet potato, Okinawan sweet potato, okra, bitter melon, corn, green papaya, fern shoots, snow peas, burdock root (gobo), breadfruit, kabocha, beans or lentils), one-half cup/day

- Konnyaku or shirataki noodles, per package portions

- Poi, one-fourth cup/day

Grains

- Low-carb tortilla, one serving
- Dave's Killer Thin-Sliced Powerseed® bread, one slice
- Steel-cut oatmeal, one-half cup, cooked
- Quinoa or brown rice, one-third cup, cooked

- Flackers Crackers (or similar low-carb cracker), one serving

For cravings, crunchy or sweet
- Pork rinds
- Cheese whisps or moon cheese
- Flackers
- Lily's dark chocolate varieties
- Dry roasted edamame
- Nori (dried packaged seaweed, one packet)
- Make your own trail mix: one-fourth cup nuts + one-eighth cup Lily's dark chocolate chips

For Instagram or website ideas
- All Day I Dream About Food
- GnomGnom Yum
- Diet Doctor

Things to watch out for:
- Tropical and nonberry fruits on a regular basis as they have high glycemic loads (see sidebar below)
- Anything sugar sweetened (cakes, cookies, juices, candy, soda, barbeque or teriyaki sauce)
- "Low-fat" products (low fat is a euphemism for high sugar)
- Hidden carbs in dressings, sauces, and premade items containing breadcrumbs (e.g., meatballs)

• FOOD *for* THOUGHT •
What is the Glycemic Load?

The glycemic load is a calculation that takes into account how high your blood glucose spikes after a meal (also known as the glycemic index (GI) of the food) and how long it *stays* high.[61]

Why is this important? Remember that when blood glucose spikes, insulin also spikes—and because insulin is one of our key fat-storage and hunger hormones, we want to keep insulin as *low* as possible.

Therefore, knowing the glycemic load for certain carbs vs. the glycemic index alone can be very useful.

Here's how to do the calculation, plus a nice example from the Glycemic Index Foundation.[62]

Glycemic load = GI x carbohydrate (g) content per portion/100.

A single apple has a GI of 38 and contains 13 grams of carbohydrate.

GL = 38 x 13/100 = 5

A white potato has a GI of 85 and contains 14 grams of carbohydrate.

GL = 85 x 14/100 = 12

We can therefore predict that the potato will have over twice the glycemic effect of an apple.

Similar to the glycemic index, the glycemic load of a food can be classified as low, medium, or high.

Low: 10 or less

Medium: 11–19

High: 20 or more

A WORD ABOUT NON-SUGAR SWEETENERS

The use of non-sugar sweeteners like Splenda, Stevia, erythritol, and monk fruit is a controversial and complex topic. I do believe these have been unfairly demonized, with many people believing that "natural sugars" are better for the body. With this, I strongly disagree.

Some data suggest that certain non-sugar sweeteners can increase insulin,[63] alter gut bacteria, which may in turn play a role in weight gain,[64] and trigger craving centers in the brain,[65] which could theoretically increase the desire for low-carb-unfriendly foods. But I believe these effects may be less significant than if actual sugar was eaten. Simply put, the use of non-sugar sweeteners, in moderation, is something that I feel is absolutely okay for my patients.

Reasonable choices that are less likely to impact insulin levels include:[66]

- Stevia
- Erythritol
- Monk fruit extract
- Xylitol
- Sucralose

Try to avoid non-sugar sweeteners that contain fillers such as dextrose or maltodextrin when possible, as these may impact blood sugar and insulin levels.

DO I NEED VITAMINS?

In order to make sure you are getting enough of several critical components while you are on a low-carb eating plan, I would generally answer yes, you need vitamins. A standard multivitamin is a great idea, since many clinical studies looking at the safety of low-carb eating plans have included supplementation with vitamins and minerals.[67] The vitamin doesn't have to be fancy—whatever is the least expensive at your regular supermarket should be fine. Your doctor may recommend specific vitamin supplements for you based on your age, sex, and medical conditions, of course. At a bare minimum, in my opinion, a good multivitamin for those on a low-carb eating plan should include sodium, magnesium, calcium, vitamin D, omega-3 fats, and zinc—but always check with your personal physician first.

SODIUM

This much-maligned mineral is critically important in our diet. Sodium helps our cells conduct nerve impulses efficiently and makes sure our muscles contract. When insulin in the body is high with metabolic syndrome, the kidneys abnormally retain too much sodium, causing bloating, leg swelling, and high blood pressure. When insulin drops (such as with a low-carb eating plan), the kidneys will release more sodium. Therefore, it's critical to consume a healthy amount of salt to avoid symptoms of lightheadedness, dizziness, and constipation (4–5 g daily is recommended). This can be accomplished by using a little extra salt on your food and drinking one to two cups of your choice of broth daily. This could be chicken, beef, or vegetable broth—just make sure it's not low-sodium broth though!

MAGNESIUM

Magnesium is also critical for nerve and muscle function, especially our heart muscle. We get it from meats, leafy greens, and nuts. Deficiencies can cause fatigue or muscle twitching and cramps. Check to see if your multivitamin includes at least 200 mg per day.

VITAMIN D

While severe vitamin D deficiency is not common in developed countries, mild deficiency is common and is associated with bone concerns like osteoporosis and increased fracture risk. Carrying excess weight also puts you at risk for deficiency.[68] Vitamin D has an inactive and an active form, and the conversion occurs in our skin in response to sunlight. The standard recommendation is for people at risk for deficiency to consume 600–800 IU of vitamin D daily. But, if you are deficient already, you may need more, so I do recommend checking with your physician on this.

OMEGA-3 FATS

Omega-3 is one of two essential fatty acids that our bodies need. The other is omega-6, but with a standard American diet, we tend to get too much of this. Omega-3 fats help to decrease our risk of coronary heart disease and are important for brain and eye health. While there are short-chain forms of omega-3 (found in leaves, algae, and seed oils), these aren't converted as efficiently to the active form needed by our bodies as the longer-chain forms (found in fish oil and seafood). You probably get enough omega-3 fatty acids if you eat fish three times weekly or eggs from chickens eating omega-3-rich feed. Another great way to get your omega-3 allowance is from capsules, one gram daily.

ZINC

Zinc deficiency can result from diabetes or if you've had any kind of weight-loss surgery. Symptoms of zinc deficiency include very dry skin, problems with skin healing, abnormal taste or smell, trouble building or maintaining muscle, and even slow weight loss. Good food sources for zinc include meats, chicken, and nuts, but if you don't eat a lot of these, check to see that your multivitamin also includes 30 mg of zinc.

• FOOD *for* THOUGHT •
Should I Track What I Eat?

Short answer: *Yes!* I highly recommend tracking at least for the first two to four weeks that you are adapting to a new way of eating.

Why track?

— Increases mindfulness of what you eat

— Helps troubleshoot any problems or concerns, especially if you are working one-on-one with a physician, dietitian, or health coach who will need to review your food choices

— Helps you learn more about nutrition

— Increases accountability to yourself

Tracking is *not* about making yourself neurotic or stressed. There are some wonderful tools and apps out there that make it easy, such as Carb Manager, MyFitnessPal, Lose It!, and Selectivor. You could also just use good old-fashioned pen and paper, too!

If this seems too difficult, here's something else you can try: simply take photos of what you eat and drink. You can create a special album on your device to store these photos for easy access. For extra accountability and reinforcement, I've had many patients post their food photos to their social media accounts, which can be a wonderful source of group support.

As we begin adapting, it becomes pretty clear that no two days are alike in our schedule. We all have incredibly busy days, and days that are a bit more low demand. I like to call these "performance days" and "recharge days."

FUELING FOR PERFORMANCE DAYS

Days with high demands on your time and energy—your busiest days—require high-performance fuels and fluids for you to be at optimal function level. On these days, you also want to minimize the chances of having a dietary slip into unhealthy habits just because you are busy.

– Keep easy snacks handy (precut or prebagged veggies or a low-glycemic-load fruit, individual cheese sticks, keto-friendly protein bars, individual nut packs, boiled eggs, protein jerky, etc.)

– When on the go or if you're grabbing quick meals out, think proteins/greens/fats with your food choices as much as you can. It's even possible at a fast-food joint—just remove buns from burgers, avoid extra sausages, and order a side salad.

FUELING FOR RECHARGE DAYS

On recharge days, we have an opportunity to kick back, relax a little, and start prepping for our next performance day. On recharge days, aim to do the following:

– Meal prep for performance days—make a list of preferred proteins/greens/fats for shopping, precut your veggies and place into bags for the week, boil eggs, etc.

– Grocery shop and perhaps try a new low-carb recipe.

– Enjoy a meal with loved ones or eat a meal in a place that represents serenity for you, perhaps out in the yard or on your balcony if you have one. You might even choose to light up your eating space with candles for a relaxing ambience!

SAMPLE WEEKS

SAMPLE WEEK 1—MODERATE LOW CARB

≤3–5 servings of extras per day (50–75 g total carbs, if you are counting)

(*Note: vegetarian proteins may be substituted for any listed meat options)

Day	Breakfast	Lunch	Snack *CAN BE INCLUDED AT ANY TIME DURING THE DAY (AS NEEDED)	Dinner
SUNDAY	One thin-slice Dave's Killer Bread or Costco Keto Bread, one-half sliced avocado mixed with lemon, salt, and pepper, and one egg, pan-fried in olive oil on top	Portobello pizza: one portobello mushroom cap, one-fourth cup zero-sugar pizza sauce, one-fourth cup shredded full-fat mozzarella cheese, sliced tomatoes, and basil	One cup plain, full-fat Greek yogurt with three-fourths cup blueberries	Grilled steak with one-half cup (cooked) baked sweet potato and cauliflower rice with olive oil, salt, and pepper
MONDAY	One-half cup cooked, unsweetened steel-cut oatmeal with one-fourth cup raspberries, dash of cinnamon, and one scoop protein powder (any flavor)	Leftover grilled steak over fresh salad greens with one-fourth cup diced tomatoes, blue cheese crumbles, and blue cheese dressing	One hard-boiled egg with salt, pepper, and paprika	Stir-fry (with soy sauce, sesame oil, and optional pinch of red chili) including one-half block firm tofu and one cup chopped eggplant with one-third cup brown rice and one cup miso soup
TUESDAY	One cup full-fat cottage cheese with one-half medium apple, sliced, one-eighth cup slivered almonds, and cinnamon	Chef salad: mixed greens, diced ham or turkey, one sliced boiled egg, 10 parmesan cheese whisps, one-fourth cup roasted red peppers, and creamy ranch dressing	One cheese stick with two mini cucumbers	Broiled salmon fillet with one cup (cooked) roasted butternut squash, kale salad with olive oil, garlic, lemon, and sprinkled parmesan cheese
WEDNESDAY	Veggie breakfast wrap with one low-carb tortilla wrap, two MorningStar Farms® sausage links, one scrambled egg, sprinkle of cheddar cheese on top, 2 tbsp guacamole, and 2 tbsp salsa (store-bought is fine)	Spring mixed greens with one-half block firm tofu, one-fourth cup kimchi, sliced cucumber and radish, one-fourth cup sliced tomatoes, with homemade Asian-style dressing (sesame oil, rice wine vinegar, stevia, soy sauce)	One Trader Joe's Norwegian Crispbread topped with a slice of smoked salmon, capers, and one sliced red onion ring	Beyond Meat Burger on two slices Costco Keto Bread topped with sprouts, lettuce, or arugula, onions, and mustard or 1 tbsp sugar-free ketchup

Day	Breakfast	Lunch	Snack	Dinner
THURSDAY	Omelet with three slices ham, spinach, mushrooms, and sprinkled cheese, plus one-half cup fried sweet potato fries in olive oil with salt, pepper, and herbs	Chicken Caesar wraps: 3 oz shredded rotisserie chicken mixed with creamy Caesar dressing, wrapped in romaine or butter lettuce leaves	One-half cup Cheese Whisps	Slow-cooker pork loin made with broth and flavored with capers and other herbs or spices, plus olive-oil-roasted Brussel sprouts
FRIDAY	Leftover roasted Brussel sprouts, with scrambled eggs	Greek salad made with cucumber, one-fourth cup tomatoes, one oz feta cheese, sliced red onion, 2 tbsp sliced green olives, and one-half cup chickpeas tossed with 2 tbsp olive oil, 2 tbsp red wine vinegar, garlic, and topped with one can sardines, drained	One slice Costco Keto Bread with 1 tbsp natural nut butter topped with three thin-sliced strawberries or 10 blueberries	Simmered chicken thighs (simmer in soy sauce, monk fruit sweetener, broth of choice, garlic, and ginger) plus sautéed riced cauliflower and steamed bok choy greens
SATURDAY	One cup full-fat plain Greek yogurt with 1 tbsp unsweetened coconut flakes and 1 tbsp slivered almonds	Chicken and vegetable "pasta": one cup cooked konjac or shirataki noodles, plus sautéed zucchini, eggplant, sun-dried tomatoes, green olives, and sliced chicken breast in olive oil	Low-carb protein bar of choice with cup of tea	Southwest salad with cooked ground meat of choice, diced tomatoes, shredded cheese, 2 tbsp guacamole, 1 tbsp sour cream, and salsa

SAMPLE WEEK— VERY LOW CARB/KETOGENIC

≤0–2 servings of extras per day (<30–40 g total carbs)

*(*Note: vegetarian proteins may be substituted for any meat options listed below.
**check "Resources" chapter for more details)*

Day	Breakfast	Lunch	Snack	Dinner
SUNDAY	Jicama wraps with one-half sliced avocado mixed with smoked salmon, sugar-free natural mayo, salt, and pepper	"Fathead" Pizza Crust, zero-sugar pizza sauce, one-fourth cup shredded mozzarella cheese, pepperoni slices, diced tomatoes, basil, and green leafy salad with vinaigrette dressing	One boiled egg with salt, pepper, and paprika	Grilled steak with one-half cup mashed cauliflower, and roasted broccoli with olive oil, salt, and pepper
MONDAY	One cup hot coffee or tea with ½ tbsp coconut oil, ½ tbsp butter or ghee, and one serving size vanilla (or any flavor) protein powder	Egg salad (made with diced boiled egg, natural mayo, and salt or pepper to taste) scooped into mini-pepper "boats" (halved mini sweet bell peppers)	One cup Two Good Greek yogurt	Stir-fry (with soy sauce, sesame oil, and chili oil to taste) one-half block firm tofu, one cup chopped eggplant with one cup riced cauliflower, and one cup miso soup
TUESDAY	Omelet with diced sausage, spinach, mushrooms, and three cherry or grape tomatoes	Chef salad with mixed greens, diced ham or turkey, one boiled egg, 10 parmesan cheese whisps, one-fourth cup roasted red peppers with mustard vinaigrette	One cheese stick with one stick celery	Broiled salmon with one cup roasted broccoli, and kale salad dressed with olive oil, garlic, lemon, and sprinkled parmesan cheese
WEDNESDAY	Veggie breakfast wrap with one low-carb fajita-size wheat tortilla wrap, two MorningStar Farm® sausage links, 2 tbsp guacamole, and 2 tbsp salsa	Mixed greens with one-half block firm tofu, one-fourth cup kimchi, sliced cucumber and radish, one-fourth cup sliced tomatoes, and nori (seaweed) with homemade Asian dressing (sesame oil, rice wine vinegar, stevia, soy sauce)	Low-carb "mug cake" with almond flour, sweetener, cocoa powder, one egg, topped with ½ tsp ChocZero dark chocolate chips	Beyond Meat Burger with two roasted portobello mushrooms (as the buns), topped with sprouts, lettuce or arugula, onions, and mustard

Day	Breakfast	Lunch	Snack	Dinner
THURSDAY	"Chaffle" waffle (made with almond flour, egg, and shredded mozzarella cheese), three sliced strawberries, ChocZero maple syrup	Chicken Caesar wraps: shredded rotisserie chicken mixed with creamy Caesar dressing, wrapped in romaine lettuce or green cabbage leaves	Three mini bell peppers stuffed with shredded cheese of choice and then baked	Baked sea bass fillets with olive-oil-roasted broccoli, cauliflower, and Brussel sprouts plus one serving of Costco Healthy Protein Noodles
FRIDAY	Leftover roasted broccoli, cauliflower, and brussels sprouts with two scrambled eggs and a sprinkle of parmesan cheese	Greek salad made with cucumber, tomatoes, crumbled feta cheese, sliced red onion, olive tapenade, and sardines	Celery sticks with 1 tbsp natural nut butter and sprinkled with 1 tbsp unsweetened coconut flakes	Hearty seafood soup with clams, mussels, squid, and shrimp simmered in vegetable broth with diced tomato and onion
SATURDAY	One cup full-fat plain Greek yogurt with sprinkle of unsweetened coconut flakes or cacao nibs, 1 tbsp natural peanut butter, and Stevia drops	Chicken and vegetable "pasta": one cup cooked konjac or shirataki noodles plus sautéed zucchini, eggplant, asparagus, sun-dried tomatoes, green olives, and sliced chicken breast sautéed in olive oil	1 tsp cream cheese and diced olives rolled into one slice salami	Southwest salad: with cooked ground beef, diced tomatoes, shredded cheese, 2 tbsp guacamole, 1 tbsp sour cream, and salsa

For more details on some of these items, including websites and recipes for items like fathead pizza, low-carb mug cake, and chaffles, please see the "Resources" chapter at the end of the book.

An important fueling note—it may feel overwhelming to some to think about a total diet overhaul in one go.

No sweat—as I have mentioned before, you can adapt in stages, step by step! For example, you can start with any of these suggestions:

— Eliminate processed sugars (sodas, cookies, sweets).

— Make one meal per day focused on protein and greens.

— Make one day per week focused on protein and greens.

— Resolve to cook one meal per week.

— Sign up for a healthy meal delivery service to assist (depending on your budget).

— Any eating goal that feels meaningful to you!

> *Patient Voice:* MW *(male, truck driver)*
>
> *"I felt so much better even just without all the soda I was drinking. It motivated me to start taking even more steps to change."*

Once you've chosen your goal of what to adapt to in terms of initial eating plans, keep in mind that later you will be able to adjust as needed and desired.

CHAPTER TAKEAWAY POINTS

Adapting to a low-carb lifestyle can begin with a focus on proteins/greens/fats as principal nutrients.

There's no "one right way" to go about eating changes, and you can even begin with changing just one meal per day or even one per week! And always work with the help and advice of your physician. Reach out to her to talk about yourself, your needs, and what is important to *you*.

SELF-EXPLORATION

What fueling goals will you aim to adapt to? Write them down:

My fueling goals:

_____

My plan for tracking my eating (app, journal, photos, etc.):

_____

6

ADAPTING TO FLOWING

"The more fluid you are, the more you are alive."
—Attributed to Arnaud Desjardins

Along with fueling your body properly in the adapt process, it's also critical to incorporate flowing—or creating lifestyle balance.

ADAPTING TO FLOWING

Creating balance in your lifestyle may be an entirely new concept for you. Many of us have the mindset of constantly giving to other people, achieving tasks, and meeting obligations, and it may feel like this is so deeply ingrained that it's part of our DNA. Unfortunately, this can not only be damaging to our mental health and well-being but it can also be a serious roadblock in the process of lifestyle change. If you have not been in the habit of devoting regular time to yourself before, flowing will be something you will have to get used to gradually.

One easy way to start: choose to earmark 10 minutes per day to work on at least one of the following flowing aims:

- Self-Reflection or gratitude

- Mindfulness

- Sleep

1. Self-Reflection or gratitude

   Assess how you are doing, each and every day. What happened in your day that stood out for you? If positive, write it down, and notice your feelings. Tell yourself, "Today I am grateful for X." Make daily gratitude your new habit. If negative, can you learn from it and let it go? For those of us who are perfectionists, this can be incredibly challenging.

2. Mindfulness

   Aim to focus on your breath for 30–60 seconds during a quiet time (waiting on a grocery store line, sitting at a traffic signal, waiting for an appointment, prior to taking your first bite of a meal, etc.). Rather than leaping out of bed in the morning and immediately starting your day with email, work, or family obligations, take five minutes to use a meditation app to focus on yourself. I'm a fan of Insight Timer, which has free guided exercises (ranging from one minute to 20+ minutes) to help declutter the brain.

   You can also try what are known as progressive muscle relaxation techniques (see: *QR: The Quieting Reflex* by Charles Stroebel, MD, PhD).[69] These techniques guide you to tense and release different muscles of the body, one after another, as you breathe and focus on the sensations. Progressive muscle relaxation practice can help us realize the areas where we hold tension, whether in the jaw, neck, shoulders, hands, or even our feet![70] Doing the exercises for the first time can be quite eye-opening as you may find areas of tension that you never imagined could be there.

Do these two flowing aims feel too time-consuming? A good way to combine both self-reflection or gratitude and mindfulness is summed up in the following well-known Zen Buddhist premeal prayer:[71]

- First: Let us reflect on our own work, and the efforts of those who brought us this food.

- Second: Let us be aware of the quality of our deeds as we receive this meal.

- Third: What is most essential is the practice of mindfulness, which helps us transcend greed, anger, and delusion.

- Fourth: In order to continue our practice for all beings, I accept this offering.

If you were to come up with your own version of a premeal reflection to help improve mindfulness, how would it read?

3. Sleep

You've probably heard this before—sleep is critical to healthy weight balance. The circadian "clock" in our bodies that controls sleep and wakefulness also helps regulate our metabolic pathways. This is why people who are chronically sleep deprived and/or those who engage in shift work, such as healthcare workers and airplane crews, have higher rates of metabolic syndrome and increased fat production in fat cells.[72] Lack of quality sleep also increases chronic inflammation, which leads to cardiovascular disease, cancers, and degenerative brain diseases.[73]

Patient Voice: *SA (male, student)*

"I am WAY hungrier when I don't sleep well."

So, if we know good sleep is healthy and important, why can it be so challenging for us to attain?

Part of the reason is likely that our society rarely encourages us to disconnect, log off, and relax. The use of smartphones and devices gives us incredible resources for information and to connect with others, but that can easily turn into a double-edged sword and become way too stimulating for our brains. Many of us turn to prescription medications to help or over-the-counter sleep aids such as melatonin or diphenhydramine (the ingredient in the allergy medication Benadryl), which provides only temporary and limited relief. Eventually, our brains will literally outsmart the drugs' effects and prevent us from sleeping well in the long term, which is why pills are not a permanent solution.

We do know that if you are tired, and you can allow yourself to completely relax mentally and physically, sleep will happen automatically. This, however, is the key: allowing yourself to relax. When we were babies and during childhood, this was an easy thing to do, but many of us in adulthood need to relearn the habit. This is where some of the apps mentioned above (such as Insight Timer) can be incredibly helpful, with wind down exercises, meditations, and sound therapy to soothe the brain.

Bud Winter addresses sleep throughout his book, *Relax and Win*.[74] His method of relaxation and sleep training was used by the US military during World War II. He taught pilots how to sleep anywhere—including to the sound of gunfire! If pilots can learn to sleep to gunfire, you can learn to sleep with the "shots" that bombard your tired brain, too.

Some tips for adapting to better sleep

- Sleep can occur when the brain is relaxed for as short a period as 10 seconds—it doesn't take hours of lying in bed to accomplish this.

- Hours of lying in bed will in fact have the opposite effect: it will condition your brain to associate your bed with wakefulness! Not something we want.

- Wait until you feel sleepy before getting into bed. If you can't sleep after 10 minutes, get out of bed and perform a light activity or read until you feel sleepy again.

- Wake up at the same time daily (even on non-workdays) and avoid napping to give your circadian clock a fast reset.

- When you wake up, expose your face to sunlight for at least 10 minutes.

- Avoid caffeine of any kind after noon. Discontinue alcohol, which is also a sleep disruptor.

- Concentrate on relaxing the eyes and speech muscles of the mouth and throat to help increase speed to sleep.

- Put devices on "do not disturb" for at least two hours prior to bedtime and turn off the TV. Looking at a screen of any kind will increase the time that it takes for you to get to sleep.

- Thinking about work or other stimulating activities or perseverating on negative thoughts will delay sleep. Consider keeping a notebook next to your bed, so that if you find yourself overthinking, you can quickly jot down your thoughts to "empty" them out of your head, so to speak.

- If you regularly use medications to help you sleep, it can take some time to learn to sleep without them, and you may need the assistance of your physician to safely discontinue use. Be patient with your body and your brain.

Journals and apps can be very helpful, not only to track your progress but to provide structured tools to guide you on achieving your flowing aims. Here are some suggestions:

Self-reflection or mindfulness apps: Insight Timer, Headspace, Breathe, Calm, 3 Minute Mindfulness. Insight Timer's free version has all kinds of different tools to help you breathe through strong emotions like anxiety and settle down for sleep. It even has live streaming yoga classes for all levels!

Sleep apps: Sleep Cycle, Relax & Sleep Well. There is also an app that combines most of the above—called WHOOP—but it is more expensive.

Alternatively, you can use a plain old notebook to give you more freedom to track your ideas and feelings in a way that comes more naturally to you.

With time, flowing practices will become habitual, and you'll feel your day is incomplete without at least one of them!

CHAPTER TAKEAWAY POINTS

Learning to flow with life's up and downs via practicing self-reflection, gratitude, and mindfulness can be just as critical as eating is to the process of adapting. Improving sleep can also greatly enhance our metabolic health and further our goals with weight loss.

SELF EXPLORATION

1. Try this exercise: set a timer on your phone for two minutes and set the phone aside. Sit up comfortably with a straight spine, and observe your breath as you inhale and exhale. Notice the pauses BETWEEN the breaths as well as the breaths themselves. How do you feel?

2. One thing I am grateful right now for is:

_____

7

HOW TO ADJUST

"Insanity is doing the same thing over and over,
and expecting a different result."
—*Unknown*

You've adapted to a new way of eating and thinking about food.

You are likely feeling better.

Your clothes may feel looser, and there may be less bloat.

Your blood pressure may have dropped a bit—if you're checking.

You may be seeing the scale start to move, too.

All great things!

Given all this, it's critical to start learning about the adjustment phase, which consists of making ongoing tweaks to respond to how your body is changing.

How will you know if you need to adjust? And why would you need to make adjustments if you've learned to eat more healthily?

The main reason to consider adjusting your eating plan is if your weight loss is slowing or if you hit a weight plateau. You may be okay with the weight plateau—perhaps it represents a new weight you feel comfortable sticking with for a while. But if you are not happy with the stoppage on the scale, read on.

WEIGHT PLATEAUS

Congratulations! Hitting a weight plateau means that you have met the number one sign that you should enter the adjustment phase.

First things first. Weight plateaus are not only common they are also a *normal* part of any lifestyle change. Completely normal. Weight loss is not a continuous process and the trajectory can be quite irregular.

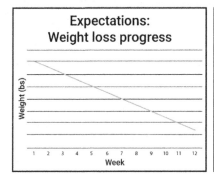
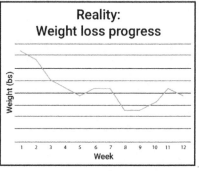

Plateaus are not a sign that your best efforts are worthless and that you should completely abandon ship. You haven't done anything wrong, and you are most certainly *not* a failure either, so please don't beat yourself up!

So, what are weight plateaus, why do they happen, and how do you know that you have hit one?

We talked about the high weight set point issue back in Chapter 3—a theory that our bodies have a biological imperative to gain and preserve fat stores—so of course it's natural that as you lose weight, your body will have periods of time where it will fight back against you in an attempt to preserve what it sees as its "normal" weight, no matter how much we may not like it. Think of weight plateaus as simply a signal that it's now time to adjust your strategies to better meet your goals. It's critical to understand that with even a 5–10-lb. loss, your body is changing rapidly, so doing the same thing over and over won't necessarily give you the same results.

Let's look at the facts.

First, are you even in a plateau? Sometimes people panic when the scale hasn't moved for a couple of days, or even a week, or when it bumps up a pound as a result of the menstrual cycle, constipation, or water retention. These are *not* actually plateaus.

Definition of a weight plateau: no change in the scale or in any body measurements (be it inches around the waist or body fat) for four weeks or longer.

If that's where you are, read on!

Here's how your body's mechanisms for reinforcing weight plateaus work.

— As you lose weight, you burn less energy: your basal metabolic rate drops, and the amount of energy you expend with daily activities will also drop as you are carrying less excess weight.[75] Think about it this way: because you carry less weight, it takes less energy to move your new, smaller body weight around. This can occur even with a loss of only five pounds.

— If you haven't been active or your protein intake is inadequate, your muscle mass may drop as well. Lower muscle mass equals lower metabolism, which equals less weight loss.

— Your energy requirements change, meaning you may need different amounts of protein/fat/carbs and calories to continue to drive the weight-loss train. As an example, let's say that you found that eating

71

three "extras" a day from Chapter 5 was enough to keep the scale moving early on from 240 to 225 lbs. However, this might not work to get you from 225 lbs. down to your 220-lb. goal weight. You may be exceeding your *new* carb threshold for weight loss.

— We have another key hunger-regulating hormone besides insulin: it's called ghrelin. This hormone is released by the stomach when empty, and its release triggers us to eat. As you lose weight, your ghrelin levels increase over time, which in turn increases your cravings and your desire to eat.[76] When this happens, your body senses danger, as it is still clinging to your high weight set point from before. So, it kicks in as many defense mechanisms as possible to try to get you back there.

— Psychologically, adjustments are needed as well. It can be fun and exciting at first to receive compliments on how your body is changing, but it can also be overwhelming and exhausting for some (more on weight maintenance in Chapter 11, "Adapting and Adjusting for Life"). You may develop the mindset that "the job is done" and become more lax with your goals to put yourself and your body first. You may feel guilty that you've paid less attention to other responsibilities while you were focusing on getting your health in order.

Things to think about when in a plateau:

— Have you relaxed your eating to allow more carbohydrates to sneak in? This can often happen if you are indulging too frequently in "keto-friendly" commercial snacks or products advertised as low carb. These carbs still count, and they will add up.

— Are you eating more frequently or grazing throughout the day? Even with low-carb eating, insulin levels will still increase in response to snacking in susceptible individuals, which can interfere with ongoing weight loss.

— Are you overeating protein or fat? Remember that weight loss happens best with both carb *and* calorie restriction, so if you overconsume energy in the form of calories, weight loss will stall. Fats contain the highest number of calories per gram of any food, so eating too-large fat portions can block the scale. How much is too much? It depends. If you keep total carbs very low (such as <20 g total/day), most people can eat at least 100 g of fat per day and still lose weight. If the carb count is higher, fat must be lower, because fats plus carbs together are also a powerful stimulus for insulin release.

— Are you drinking alcohol? Even if you drink zero-carb spirits, for some people alcohol inhibits the liver's ability to burn fat. Our liver can carry out fat oxidation very efficiently, except when it senses the presence of a toxin such as alcohol in the bloodstream. The liver will then turn its energies to removal of the toxin, which could mean stalling fat loss.

— How are your physical activity levels? Exercise can improve motivation to stay on track and lift energy levels. It also improves sleep quality, which is critical to keeping the scale moving.

— Medications: be aware of all prescription and over the counter items you use. Some medications could inadvertently be affecting your weight (refer to Chapter 4 for more on this).

How to adjust:

1. Start or restart tracking your food intake. This will give you an idea of what is working or not working for you and where there are opportunities to adjust. Are hidden starches sneaking into your eating? Have you been eating a lot of takeout that may contain hidden sugars in sauces and dressings? Are you engaging in mindless grazing due to higher stress levels? (This happens to *all* of us if we are not careful!) Refer back to Chapter 5 for tips and resources on tracking.

2. Consider reducing your carbohydrate intake. If you are consistent-
    ly eating even slightly over your daily carb tolerance, weight loss
    will immediately stall, per above. Even a small adjustment may be
    enough to get the scale moving for you again.

3. If you drink alcohol, consider stopping for one week. If that's easy, try
    to stop for two weeks or even a month. You don't have to drink a lot
    of beer, wine, or liquor for it to have an impact on your weight-loss
    efforts—even one drink a week can interrupt the process for sensitive
    individuals and particularly for women. Alcoholic drinks can add carbs
    and sugar to your daily intake. Drinking alcohol can also be dehydrat-
    ing and slow down the liver's fat-burning abilities, as discussed above.
    If that's not reason enough, alcohol also tends to disinhibit our
    self-control over what we eat, which can lead to overindulgences.
    You'll have far less restraint when faced with temptations when alco-
    hol is on board, and the guilt and shame you'll inevitably feel after-
    wards will interfere with ongoing motivation to make adjustments.
    Not worth it!

4. Consider intermittent fasting (IF) or time-restricted eating (TRE).
    IF and TRE are excellent ways to further reduce hyperinsulinemia
    on a low-carb eating plan and may help kick-start weight loss that
    has stalled.[77] Intermittent fasting can be a terrific adjustment that is
    quite simple to make, doesn't require purchasing any special food or
    products, and is totally customizable.

    There are many, many ways to fast, including weekly 24-hour fasts,
    alternate day fasting, or "OMAD" (one meal a day) types of fasting.
    Some individuals are proponents of even longer fasting, for any-
    where between three and seven days! Personally, I don't advise my
    patients to do long fasts, as there may be medical reasons not to,
    plus you can easily get the benefits from shorter, more intermittent
    fasting periods. For example, one eating pattern known as a 12:8
    hour fasting/eating ratio is generally easy for most people to adjust
    to. To do this, you would fast for 12 hours per day, and confine

your eating window to an eight-hour period. This is easiest for most people to accomplish by eating dinner by 6 p.m. and then waiting until 10 a.m. the following day to eat breakfast. Fasting is way too large a topic to discuss here, but a great resource for further reading is Dr. Jason Fung's book *The Obesity Code*.[78] If you do consider fasting, hydration and mineral replenishment is *key* (see Keto Flu in the "Speedbumps and Roadblocks" chapter). I also recommend a daily multivitamin to anyone who fasts regularly.

5. The use of meal replacements can be a highly effective adjustment to boost weight loss. I generally advise meal replacements where fasting may not be advisable or perhaps when someone is struggling with time and a busy schedule that interferes with making the healthiest choices. Low-carb meal replacements, with or without associated online coaching, can really come to the rescue here. You can simply substitute one to two meals daily with a meal replacement you enjoy. When looking for a meal replacement, try to find shakes that contain <2 g of carbohydrate per serving or bars with <5 g net per serving. Acceptable brands include Premier Protein, Adapt Your Life bars, Atkins products, Muscle Milk, Isopure, and the Vega Protein & Greens range, among many others. In terms of which meal is best to swap out for a substitute, it really depends. Many of us rush around to begin work in the morning, so the use of a meal replacement shake for breakfast works well. If you typically have a busy evening or work late, substituting a meal replacement for dinner might suit you better—it's completely up to you. You can even consider a more comprehensive meal replacement program that includes coaching and monitoring your lifestyle, such as the Ideal Protein weight-loss method.

6. Check back in with your flowing goals: do these need adjustments? Are your mood, stress, and sleep helping or not helping you? Do you feel well rested when you wake? If not, elevated levels of the hormone cortisol could be blocking your weight loss.

a. If extreme personal stress is a factor, counseling or psychotherapy may be helpful. Look to resources such as Psychologytoday.com to find a qualified psychotherapist near you. A type of psychotherapy called cognitive behavioral therapy (CBT) can do wonders to help you adjust your outlook and reduce stress.

b. If you are not active, you can start walking or doing chair exercise. If you don't feel comfortable with in person group exercise, a yoga class on YouTube can be a great option. You can even set a calendar reminder to dance around your living room for 10 minutes a day (minimum) as a work break—this is one of my personal favorites!

c. Don't forget mindfulness and gratitude. Check out Tinybuddha.com for some daily inspirational quotes to give you a boost. Stepping away from the laptop for just five minutes and breathing fresh air outdoors can help renew you in surprising ways. We are often so critical of ourselves. Try to find one thing you love about your body (it could be anything—your hair, the curve of your hips, your eye color, even your fingernails) and express gratitude for this to someone, anyone—even to yourself in the mirror.

7. If you qualify, consider discussing the use of weight-loss medications with your physician. More about this in the "Turbo Boosters for Adjustments" chapter coming up.

8. And finally, remind yourself that your health still comes first at all times. This is critical. Perpetually putting your own needs last because of guilt or any other reason is never justified. You can't take care of the world if you don't take care of yourself first and foremost.

Here's something to think about as well: you may actually still be losing weight. It's just that it's going very slowly. We all have high expectations, but it's important to remember that weight loss tends not to happen in a linear fashion. You might lose three to six pounds one month, then only one pound the next, or you may even gain a pound. This is common and 100% normal, even when your eating and lifestyle are perfectly on point. Although you might not be seeing changes on the scale, keep tracking what you eat and stick to your plan. Trust that your body is still doing its work.

Overall, try not to get too upset or be too hard on yourself. Having to make adjustments is a totally normal part of the weight-loss process. After all, weight gain is a natural process for the body. It's common to become angry or frustrated or to start beating yourself up. But if you approach the problem more like a detective and look at yourself like a curious observer or a kind friend, you'll have a much better chance of long-term success.

CHAPTER TAKEAWAY POINTS

Needing to make adjustments to your lifestyle plan is a sure sign that your body is changing for the better. Learning to adjust will help create a new set of skills that will greatly enhance your ability to improve your health for life.

SELF-EXPLORATION

Adjustments I'd like to consider making:

Fueling:

_____

Flowing:

_____

8

SPEEDBUMPS AND ROADBLOCKS: MORE OPPORTUNITIES TO ADJUST

"Sometimes when things are falling apart, they may actually be falling into place."
—Unknown

It's inevitable that obstacles will occur along the road to better health.

Dr. Kevin Snyder, international best-selling author, keynote speaker, and blogger, created this doodle which I think sums this idea up perfectly:[79]

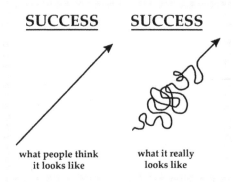

I like to think of each of these squiggles as an area where an adjustment happened so progress could continue along the path.

Let's take a look at some of the most common concerns people encounter when transitioning to a lower-carb eating plan and how to make adjustments.

1. Keto "Flu"

    Ahh the dreaded keto flu. If your body is accustomed to eating large amounts of sugars and simple starches, symptoms such as lightheadedness, unusual fatigue, nausea, headaches and muscle cramps can be common on a low-carb eating plan and can derail even the most dedicated dieter.[80] However, I want to emphasize that despite the name, you do not actually get "the flu" from reducing carbohydrates!

    Keto flu seems to occur frequently in those who consider themselves to be "social media dieters" (following whoever online is most popular, regardless of their credentials) and those who believe the key to doing a ketogenic diet is simply to cut carbs. Many see keto flu as an inevitable part of a low-carb lifestyle change.

    What actually causes keto flu or low-carb flu? Fluid and electrolyte imbalances, plain and simple. Not enough water, salt, or minerals like potassium, magnesium, and calcium can lead to all of the above symptoms.

    How to adjust: increase free fluids to 80–100 oz daily. If you drink caffeinated drinks such as coffee or tea, these can act as diuretics, so it's important to drink an extra glass of water for every caffeinated drink you have. And importantly, don't forget the salt. You'll be aiming for 4–5 g of sodium in the diet daily. Yes, that's a lot of salt, and you need it! Two cups of bouillon broth or another salty soup will generally do the trick.[81] Review Chapter 4 if you need a refresher on the importance of sodium.

Remember: keto flu is, in general, caused by poor implementation of a low-carb eating plan and can be minimized with the right adjustments, or even mostly avoided.

2. Food Cravings

Odd food cravings can pop up at any time along your path. They can be triggered by seeing certain foods—like doughnuts at the office breakfast potluck—or by social situations, stress, fatigue, and emotions, too.

I often hear people wonder if their cravings are predominantly due to "physical" hunger or "emotional" causes: is the craving physically from the stomach, or emotionally, as in a desire to feel satisfied? In a nutshell, the answer is: *both*.

We've talked quite a bit about the hormone insulin and its role in driving the hunger and fat-storage cycle. If you have metabolic syndrome, your insulin levels will be higher than normal to begin with. Add in a diet rich in starch and/or sugar and insulin levels will get bumped even higher. High insulin levels lead to a lot of hunger and cravings, often paradoxically and frustratingly, just an hour or two after you eat. What happens after that? We eat more carbohydrates and sugar, a high-insulin state is reinforced, and the vicious cycle continues.

Sugars do something else to reinforce cravings: ingestion causes activation of pleasure centers in the brain, and the feel-good chemical dopamine is released.[82] Our brains literally become addicted to the sugar in the same way they can become addicted to cocaine!

There's more to the story than just insulin. Remember the hormone ghrelin, released by the stomach when it's empty to signal to the brain that we are hungry? Turns out, ghrelin has an opposing hormone, leptin, which is released from fat cells and signals the brain that we are full.

Interestingly, when insulin is elevated due to a high-sugar diet, besides causing cravings in itself, it also causes the brain to be *less* sensitive to leptin, which will also make us feel constantly hungry.[83] There are even very rare genetic disorders of obesity where individuals have deficits in how leptin signals the brain, and guess what their primary symptom is? You guessed it: constant hunger.[84]

Remember that the pathways in our body that regulate hunger are complex and well reinforced in the body and brain. It was likely a matter of survival in cave-people times. Humans depended on their ability to find food and store energy, which wasn't always easy (hunting antelope is a lot more difficult than pulling up to the drive-through).

Understanding this can help us to see that our bodies' drive to maintain our weight is primal. Have you ever tried to lose weight by simply cutting calories and exercising more? I bet I know what happened: you probably experienced intense hunger and cravings because of the above.

No matter how much willpower you might have, eventually the body will win. Our cravings are just that powerful. Fighting cravings can feel incredibly tiring and discouraging without the right approach—we have to be smart in how we fight them.

SO HOW DO WE ADJUST?

We may have been told that cravings (not true hunger) are a signal that the body "needs" the item we are craving. Per the explanation above, you can see how this is not the case! The best way to eliminate cravings is to practice not giving in to them. How does this work?

— Keep carbohydrates low, which will drop insulin levels and improve our brains' sensitivity to leptin.

— Focus on eating proteins/greens/fats, which will help keep you full.

— Use "carb swaps" to deal with cravings: for example, rather than eating rice, use riced cauliflower. Instead of store-shelf brownies, opt for a low-carb, sugar-free recipe—there are many to be found on the Internet. Refer to the "Resources" chapter for more on these.

> **Patient Voice:** *SA (male, student)*
>
> *"It's amazing how much I craved carbs when I first started cutting down. I knew even looking at a potato chip, or a bowl of rice, would throw me off. But it's changed so much now, and I no longer feel 'addicted' to the carbs like before."*

This may sound easier said than done. But over time, as your pancreas makes less insulin and your brain re-wires itself *not* to expect constant sugar, the cravings will gradually subside. Your brain will forget the dopamine high from sugar, and the cravings will diminish. Trust me, they will eventually be gone.

3. Low Motivation or "Diet Fatigue"

Yes, you can get sick of trying to be healthy all the time. That's especially true around the holidays or other celebratory events and can be a big thing in times of stress.

It's a fact that motivation waxes and wanes over time. But even if you accept this fact, it can still be very discouraging to notice yourself caring less and less about a bite of a cookie here and there or a nibble on your kid's french fries.

I've also seen motivation wane when a patient feels resistant to embracing their own carb intolerance. We might look at a very thin person eating pizza and doughnuts and feel despondent that just looking at dinner rolls seems to cause a five-pound weight gain. An "It's not fair, why me?" type of mentality can result from this.

How to fix flagging motivation:

- Go back to your *why*. Remember how much time we spent on this in Chapter 2? It was for *exactly* this reason. Reminding yourself about *why* you embarked on this journey in the first place is a powerful tool to help get you back on track.

- Embrace your own carbohydrate-tolerance level. Yes, you might wish you had the type of metabolism where you can simply eat anything you want and not suffer any ill effects but wishing won't make you healthier. Choose to stand in *your* power, the power that you have when armed with the knowledge of how your body works. This will help you accept who you are and what you are made of and help you make the best possible choices to care for yourself.

- Get active. People who commit to even a small amount of exercise daily (like 10 minutes of walking, chair exercise, or a 10-minute YouTube workout video) have higher motivation levels than those who do not.

- De-stress. Are you overcommitted or overscheduled in other areas of your life? Feeling overwhelmed greatly affects the energy you are prepared to invest in your lifestyle changes. Cancel any nonurgent obligations and schedule one to two hours per week on your calendar just for yourself. Whether it's watching a favorite Netflix show, going out for coffee or a walk in a serene place by yourself, or just taking a nap, schedule it in!

- Mix up your eating. Sometimes motivation can wane when we feel bored with what we are eating. Fortunately, there are some amazing websites and social media channels that make low-carb and keto eating exciting and fun. I love Low Carb Yum and Diet Doctor especially. See the resources section at the end of this book for others, too.

- Find a support group. Even if your schedule is packed, finding a community of like-minded people can be key. Maybe you have coworkers or other family members who are also working on their health. Social media and online forums can be a good place to find supportive people, too. Just be aware that social media may not be confidential, and it's not a great place to find medical advice.

- Consider counseling. If low motivation is due to an extreme amount of personal stress, talk to someone. Often times employers have employee assistance programs (EAP) to provide free counseling, or you can seek out a private therapist as well. The website Psychology Today (https://www.psychologytoday.com) has local listings in all areas. If you live in a remote area (or are just busy), try online services such as PlushCare.[85] Without addressing stress or a crisis in your life, there's just no way you'll be able to commit time and energy to yourself.

4. Social Eating Issues

Have you ever struggled to say "No" at family gatherings and other social events when you are offered food that you know is not good for your body or goes against your health goals?

It's a fact that even when loved ones know you are trying to lose weight and get healthier, you often feel pressured to make a bad choice, have seconds, or eat dessert.

This doesn't necessarily mean that others want to sabotage you or ruin your success— it can just be because of history, culture, and a habit of food being a gift to share with those you love.

We were able to avoid the bulk of these situations during the COVID-19 pandemic. At the time of this book's writing, vaccines are now becoming more widely available, so I expect social gatherings will increasingly become the norm again.

Here are some things you can say when you're with others and are offered something you don't want to eat so you can stay on track with your wellness goals:

If you are in an environment where you feel comfortable sharing:

- "I can't, unfortunately. I'm committed to sticking with my health journey right now."

- "I have _____ (carbohydrate intolerance, high cholesterol, prediabetes, etc.), so I'm making changes in what I eat to improve my health."

If you prefer to be more indirect:

- "No, thank you." (Simple and polite, no explanation needed.)

- "I sure wish I could have some!"

- "Thanks, but I'm so full from all the other delicious food right now. Maybe a little later."

- "Thanks, I'll pass and just keep you company while you enjoy!"

If offered seconds:

- "No, thank you. It was delicious. Can I have the recipe?"

- "No, thanks. Hey, how are your kids doing—I haven't seen them lately!" (Diversion tactic!)

- "You know, I realized that my stomach doesn't feel good when I eat _____, so now I try to avoid feeling like that."

- "My doctor told me I can't eat that. But it smells amazing!"

If you feel a need to explain or are pushed further, you can say, "Sorry, that just doesn't agree with me," or "Sorry, I need to choose what I eat more carefully for my health."

Rarely, some people may take your refusal personally and say something like, "Well, I eat cake every day, and I'm fine." Just consider such a moment as a great opportunity for you to focus on yourself and putting your needs and goals first!

Patient Voice: *JS (female, sales associate)*

"I grew up without much, and I think my parents showed love for us by feeding us as much as we wanted so we wouldn't feel poor. I gained weight from early on and developed diabetes, high blood pressure, and sleep apnea. I had to face the choice of getting sicker vs. having that difficult conversation. That was so hard to do, but once they realized that the food was hurting me, they were willing to change. I had to teach my family that there are other ways to show love than by buying tons of junk."

5. Travel

   Travel can be tough enough without also facing the challenge of food choices. Even the most perfectly planned trip can be stressful, especially at the time of writing due to extra pandemic precautions and restrictions but also because of canceled flights, traffic delays, or getting lost. You've made the commitment to eat healthier, and you don't want travel to derail your plans. How can you adjust to reduce the stress of finding something healthy to eat in unfamiliar locations and situations?

a.   Prepare—*before* you leave home.

Many of us fall into the mindset of being a hostage to unhealthy temptations on the road. This is false! You can make smart choices on how, when, and what you eat. All it takes is a little bit of preparation.

Most modes of travel allow you to bring your own food or snacks. So why get stuck paying five dollars for that small canister of potato chips on the airplane? If you prepare, when that small urge of hunger hits you, you won't be tempted to buy junk food, and you'll have something more manageable and healthier on hand. Easy travel snacks that are great for a roadside stop on a long car trip include one-fourth cup of nuts in small baggies, hard-boiled eggs, cut veggies, or low-sugar protein bars. If you don't have food handy and are looking for a place to stop, skip fast-food joints whenever possible and look for an open-air market or a small grocery store, as these are more likely to have healthier choices. For air travel, bring an empty water bottle to fill prior to boarding, so you won't be tempted to drink high-sugar juices or sodas in flight.

Before leaving for your trip, you can also scope out the food scene at your destination. Most restaurants have their menus available online, so it's a lot easier to identify establishments with healthier fare that fits your eating goals.

If you're traveling to visit family or friends, make sure to be open about your goals ahead of time so they have an opportunity to support you as well. Supply as much of your own food as you can by grocery shopping once you arrive. You don't need a kitchen, either—many stores have grab-and-go items that will work.

b.   Keep it simple.

Sticking to the basics can help you to keep your goals front of mind and stop you from becoming overwhelmed. Most restaurants and grocery stores will have some kind of protein source and vegetables or salad greens available. Ask for plain oil and vinegar dressings and avoid the heavy sweet sauces and excess starches. Look for cafés where you can get a large salad with protein or a healthy soup instead of a heavy sub sandwich and fries.

c.   Ask for what you want.

When dining out, don't be afraid or feel intimidated to ask for healthier modifications. Most restaurants will be accommodating since they want your business. If you don't see anything on the menu that you want, ask politely for something different! Most chefs are happy to grill a simple protein for you and add a salad or vegetables on the side with a savory dressing. If you see an ingredient on the menu under a different order, then it's available in the kitchen, so just ask for it. It's important to learn to be assertive—if you don't stand up for your own body, then who will? Also, when you assert yourself, you avoid the dreaded feeling of guilt or self-defeat later.

Traveling with loved ones or colleagues can be especially challenging. They may want to treat you to a meal but then don't give you any say in dining choices. If this is the case, again, try explaining before the trip why you're committed to a healthier lifestyle. The more that people understand why you're making the choices you are, the more likely they'll be to support them.

d.   Move past slip-ups and, most of all, enjoy yourself!

Even when you try your best, sometimes, inevitably, you will go off plan. If you do, it's important not to spend time beating yourself up. Just get right back on track. Acknowledge you did the best you could under the circumstances and then determine to make the next choice a better one. Don't allow, "I blew it," or all-or-none thinking to completely derail you.

Patient Voice: *LR (female, shop owner)*

"I've been able to realize that one small mistake doesn't have to ruin all the hard work I've been doing. I notice how bad the junk food feels in my body and tell myself that I know I don't want to feel that way again!"

Remember, travel is meant to be an enjoyable, fun experience. Before you leave for your trip think of all the ways that you can have a great time that don't necessarily involve food. You can go hiking, biking, or walk to explore your new area; visit a museum, gallery, or other local attraction; or take a fitness class in a different city, which can be fun and lead you to make new friends, too. Social media can also be a great way to help you stay healthy in a different location if you meet up with people you chat with online with similar health interests. If you're visiting loved ones, focus on quality time together. Do the best you can and make the most of your experience! Happy travels.

• FOOD *for* THOUGHT •
Meal and Snack Tips on the Go

– Nuts are an excellent snack to help quench hunger, as they're packed with protein, fiber, and fat. Plus, they don't melt in the heat, expire too quickly, or crush easily. You can buy nuts (but not "trail mix," which in general is loaded with sugar) in bulk at a warehouse club store. Partition one-fourth cup of nuts into small snack bags. Keep one in your car or purse and pack an extra two in luggage.

— Green tea has antioxidant health benefits, plus it can help reduce hunger and give you a nice energy kick. Many store-bought green teas contain sugar, and it's best not to rely on the convenience store, airline, or hotel to have pure green tea—bring an extra bag (or two) to enjoy en route.

— Small, full-fat hard cheeses such as cheddar, Swiss, or muenster are filling and satisfying. Freezing them beforehand will make them last much longer, too. Individually wrapped cheeses are available at most grocery stores and warehouse clubs. Also, you can pack shredded cheeses into a small plastic bag to bring for your salad or low-carb tortilla wraps. It's a great cushioning item and easy to consume on the go.

— Boiled eggs are an omega-3-rich, protein-filled boost. Keeping them in the shell gives them extra shelf life for travel (a few hours). Bring along a bag for discarding shells conveniently after peeling.

— It's often easier to find proteins than fresh veggies on the road. To make sure you always have some available, save sealable food containers and fill with salad greens before your trip, then top with whatever protein choice is available, whether that's seafood, steak, chicken, or even a burger that you simply remove from the bun. You can also buy a large bag of greens at the grocery store when you get to your destination and partition these into smaller plastic bags, giving you a readily available supply. This also helps save money—grab-and-go can get a little pricey after a while.

— Don't forget low-carb protein bars (look for those containing ≤5 g net carbs) and meat jerkies made without sugars.

— Dehydration can tax our bodies during travel, especially air travel. Be sure to carry empty water bottles and fill prior to boarding. If you are someone who needs a little extra encouragement to drink water, sprinkle sugar-free electrolyte powder into the bottles; that way, when you fill them, you have your own instant great-tasting electrolyte drink! And, if you're like me and have a "collection" of sports drink mixer bottles (the ones with the metal mixer ball inside), just bring one of them instead. They're much easier to refill and to add the electrolytes into.

— Put your favorite low-carb salad dressing, or plain balsamic vinaigrette, into a small squeezable container or a cleaned, empty travel saline bottle (remember, it must be under 3.5 oz or 100 ml). That way you can easily pack it with your other spillable items (like toiletries) and use it on the salad you just packed.

— Use collapsible food containers to pack your food. I'm an avid recycler, and a good friend of our family gave us some collapsible silicon containers as a gift. I love them! And they're easy to pack away once everything is consumed.

— Be creative! You'd be surprised how innovative you can get even with limited resources. For example, did you know you can use tomato juice (or spicy tomato juice) in lieu of marinara sauce? Or you can add a pinch of your favorite spice flavoring to a small container of shelf-stable heavy cream to create a delicious alfredo sauce. Go ahead—experiment!

6. Cholesterol changes

Some people worry about cholesterol levels or potential changes in cholesterol levels on low-carb eating plans. Let's dissect.

There is a lot of concern, and unfair hype, in my opinion, about cholesterol and its relationship to heart attacks and strokes. We've been led to believe that total levels of cholesterol in the body are strong predictors of disease. And although it is true that our lifestyles and eating play a role in how our cholesterol levels look and the impact of cholesterol levels on disease, it may not be in the way we have learned.

As it turns out, the total cholesterol level—as commonly reported in our blood test results—is, overall, *not* a great predictor of whether we will develop heart disease. In fact, cholesterol has an important role in the body as the building blocks of all our cell membranes. Here is what's important in how cholesterol influences the risk of heart disease: (1) *how* the cholesterol is distributed—i.e., is it in the wrong places—and (2) whether inflammation is present at high levels in the body. Inflammation, in turn, will determine how the cholesterol is distributed.

• FOOD *for* THOUGHT •
Does Eating Fat Raise Blood Fat Levels?

We've also been told that eating fat raises blood cholesterol, which is only partly true.

On a low-carb eating plan, eating fat actually tends to *decrease* blood cholesterol. This is because saturated fats are burned quickly and little accumulates in the blood.[86]

Let's talk about blood cholesterol markers and common interpretations of lab test results.

    a.   High-density lipoprotein (HDL): historically known as "good cholesterol."[87] The HDL particles in the blood carry cholesterol away from cells and back to the liver where it gets broken down and passed out of the body.

    b.   Low-density lipoprotein (LDL): historically known as "bad cholesterol."[88] The LDL carries cholesterol in the blood stream to cells. However, we are now learning that there are multiple types of LDL particles, some of which may be "bad" and some of which may in fact be "good" or "better." You heard me right: LDL is not just the "bad cholesterol" as we've been told. LDL cholesterol is an entire spectrum of different-sized particles.[89] Large LDL particles are not felt to be dangerous as they are not atherogenic. This means that they are unlikely to build up or accumulate in the heart's arteries to cause disease. However, small LDL particles are still felt to be more of a concern for the heart.[90]

c. Triglycerides: circulating lipid particles that store unused sugars. High concentrations of triglycerides are a major risk factor for heart disease and stroke.

d. Total cholesterol: the sum of all the cholesterol particles in the bloodstream.

Typically, with a low-carb eating plan, blood tests show favorable changes in blood cholesterol: decreases in triglycerides and increases in high-density lipoprotein, or HDL, (which we know are protective) are extremely common. These are desirable outcomes and often result in people being able to reduce or eliminate medications designed to control high triglyceride levels.

But what about low-density lipoprotein or LDL? Here is where things get tricky, and that's because LDL is a bit harder to predict. Often it will drop with low-carb eating, but in some cases, we see it rise.

Is this a problem? Short answer: most likely, no.

Here's the somewhat longer answer, my own opinion, and my advice on how to adjust.

Potential factors influencing LDL levels on a low-carb eating plan:

1. Increased mobilization of LDL into the bloodstream due to shrinkage or breakdown of fat stores—basically, your LDL can look artificially and temporarily elevated during active weight loss.[91] Once your weight stabilizes, the LDL will stabilize.

   a. *How to adjust*: simply hold off on checking your cholesterol until three months into weight maintenance.

2. The types of LDL in your bloodstream may change. Per above, not all LDL is "bad" cholesterol—only the little ones! Typical changes seen with low-carb eating include a shift from the small, dense, more dangerous LDL particles to the larger particles, which do not seem to carry the same cardiovascular risk.[92]

   a. *How to adjust*: there's generally no need to adjust much of what you are doing for lifestyle changes. While exercise doesn't help much for the weight-loss process, as we discussed, it can promote favorable lipid balance, so if you aren't yet active, now is a good time to think about it (see Chapter 9). In addition, given that standard blood lipid testing really doesn't measure a true LDL value (it's actually a calculated value) and it tells us nothing about the LDL particle number or particle size, it may be a good idea to do an advanced lipoprotein blood test so you can learn more about the types of particles making up your LDL. Ask your physician if this type of test may be helpful. Per above, it's probably important to wait and test your lipids once your weight has been stable for several months. See the next Food For Thought section for the types of specific LDL testing available at different nationwide labs.

• FOOD *for* THOUGHT •
Beyond the LDL Alone

Test panel names that your doctor may order that include the LDL particle fractionation test (available at different clinical labs in the USA):

Quest—Advanced Lipid Profile/Cardio IQ

LabCorp—NMR LipoProfile

Diagnostic Laboratory Services—Cardio IQ Advanced Lipoprotein Profile

BioReference Laboratories—Lipoprotein Particle Evaluation

In summary: in patients following a low-carb eating plan, many favorable changes occur in the blood that indicate reduced cardiovascular risk. These include reduced blood sugars, blood pressure, and reduced markers of inflammation. If you are actively losing weight and improving your health, it wouldn't really make sense to panic about an increased LDL and start lipid-lowering drugs. Chances are good that your LDL changes will be favorable and that your LDL value will stabilize as your weight does.

Added to that, even if your LDL is high, there are other blood markers of cardiac disease that may be important in interpreting your LDL in context of what else is going on in the bloodstream. Unlike the diet–heart hypothesis mentioned in Chapter 3, current thinking is that the true trigger for cardiovascular disease development is chronic inflammation. This can be measured by a host of other lab markers (see the next Food For Thought section). If I have a patient with an isolated elevated LDL, with optimal triglycerides and HDL from doing low carb, and low levels of some of the markers of inflammation that I've listed, my level of concern goes *way* down. And how's this for another great benefit of low carb: within just two weeks of low-carb eating, you can actually improve elevated inflammatory markers![93]

• FOOD *for* THOUGHT •
Additional Markers of Inflammation Potentially Important in Cardiovascular Disease Development

High-sensitivity C-reactive protein (hs-CRP)

Homocysteine

Lp-PLA2 (PLAC test)

Myeloperoxidase

F2-isoprostanes

Ox-LDL or Oxidized lipoprotein

In summary: cholesterol interpretation can be quite complicated for those doing low carb, and every situation is different. If you have concerns about your cholesterol, I recommend a discussion with your personal physician.

• FOOD *for* THOUGHT •
The Lean Mass Hyper-Responder

There is a subset of lean and otherwise healthy individuals who experience dramatic LDL cholesterol elevations on keto—sometimes in the 2–300 mg/dL range! Other features of their cholesterol profile include low triglycerides and high HDL. Lean mass hyper-responders tend to be of normal weight, active, athletic, and free of typical signs of metabolic disease such as high blood pressure or abnormal glucose. There is not a lot we understand about these individuals' bodies, but active research is ongoing at the time of writing.

So, to recap, whether or not the LDL particles you have in the blood represent a concern depends on exactly which type they are. Fortunately, ketogenic diets tend to increase the number of large LDL particles and decrease the small LDL particles, so as previously discussed, that's likely a good thing.

8. Emotional or Stress Eating

> **Patient Voice:** SS (female, retired)
>
> *"The sweets in my mouth are soothing when I am anxious or stressed. Eating comforts me and helps me to relax."*

As you've adapted and are beginning to adjust your eating habits, it may become clear that other things are driving your eating besides just hunger. You may notice that feelings of sadness, anxiety, or stress are big eating triggers for you. Strong feelings can certainly come at inconvenient times, such as when we feel the weakest emotionally. And throughout the COVID-19 pandemic era, we've all experienced a *lot* more of these emotions than normal, making this an extra big influence and extra difficult to deal with. With emotional eating, people typically crave excess high-carb sweets or salty snacks—it's rare to see someone want to eat extra protein.

Why is emotional eating so problematic? Besides the fact that it leads to irregular eating habits, increased amounts of food eaten, and worsening of insulin resistance, it can also lead to incredible feelings of guilt, shame, and self-defeat. We don't need these extra feelings to throw us further off course. If this resonates with you, here's how to adjust.

- Given that emotional eating habits develop to help us self-soothe through difficult feelings, try to think of other ways to soothe yourself that don't involve food. Perhaps a hot bath, watching a favorite TV show, buying yourself a small gift to acknowledge your efforts, or even allowing yourself an extra hour of sleep one day can all help.

- Tame stress by practicing deep breathing, meditation, or yoga. The Insight Timer app is a fabulous tool to help you get started. The free version works great.

- Avoid boredom by distracting yourself—call a friend, browse favorite nonfood websites, play a video game, or take a quick walk.

- Forgive yourself if you go offtrack. We are all human—beating yourself up about your mistakes will only worsen the emotional eating cycle. Learn from what happened, forgive yourself, and move on.

- Talk to your doctor about weight-loss medications if you qualify. (See the chapter on "Turbo Boosters for Adjustments" for more on this subject.) Weight-loss prescriptions can help reduce emotional as well as physical hunger and cravings.

- Dr. Anita Johnston, psychologist, author, and eating disorder specialist, is a fantastic resource for addressing all sorts of emotional eating including more serious types of eating disorders. I highly recommend her work.[94]

— Seek out psychotherapy: for many of us, emotional eating is so deep seated that we need clinical support to help process and redirect our feelings. Psychotherapy will give you the best possible chance of a complete recovery and, importantly, freedom from emotional eating.

Patient Voice: *MW (female, executive)*

"I'm no longer just jumping to the snacks for relief of my stress. I've found ways to catch myself and redirect to a better way to process my feelings."

CHAPTER TAKEAWAY POINTS

Speedbumps and roadblocks are further opportunities to learn about your body and yourself and, with support and assistance, can absolutely be overcome.

9

MOVEMENT

"You can't stop the waves, but you can learn to surf."
—Jon Kabat-Zinn[95]

In this chapter, we'll discuss movement (otherwise known as exercise), which is an important part of our adapt and adjust strategy.

I also hope this chapter answers a key question that some of you may have about exercise:

"Why do I work my tail off at the gym and still not lose any weight?"

Answer: Because exercise does not actually cause weight loss on its own.

I repeat: Exercise alone does not generally lead to weight loss.

Don't get me wrong: movement does many wonderful things for our body! It increases muscle tone, improves cardiovascular fitness, decreases blood pressure,[96] and improves mood and energy.[97] Exercise also does something that most medications have not been proven to do: it helps us live longer. One study revealed that as little as 15 minutes per day of moderate exercise can extend a lifespan by three years.[98] So without a doubt exercise is an important tool for overall health and wellness.

But it absolutely, unequivocally, does not make you skinny. So why do I suggest it as part of my adapt and adjust strategy?

One of the biggest reasons is that exercise doesn't speed up your metabolism as textbooks and personal trainers often state. It actually slows metabolism! And this has been found to be especially true for those who carry excess weight. Let's break this down.

Under the "calories in, calories out" theory of exercise for weight loss, one pound of fat yields 3,500 calories of energy. So, to lose one pound of fat, we must burn 3,500 calories.

Therefore, assuming you're an average-sized person, you would need to run about 350 miles to burn off 10 lbs. of body fat (assuming that your appetite doesn't increase from all that running around).

However, studies have shown that if you suffer from obesity, with exercise your resting metabolism can *slow* as much as 5%–10%,[99] resulting in a *far lower calorie burn than expected*. Instead of losing those 10 lbs., studies have shown that those with excess weight may lose only 2–3 lbs. with the same amount of exercise.[100, 101]

Besides this metabolic drop, it's also common sense that once you start exercising, another thing happens that can counteract your weight-loss attempts: you become *hungrier*. And when you get hungrier, you eat more, often rationalizing your increased consumption with the thought of, "Well, it's okay, I'm burning the food off with exercise."

But that is not as easy as it sounds: remember, you're looking at about 350 miles of running or other intensive exercise to burn off 10 lbs. That's an awful lot! Even if you ran five miles weekly, you'd be looking at 70 weeks, or nearly a year and a half, to lose 10 lbs. by running alone. I don't know about you, but I'd sure prefer to see quicker results than that.

In addition, a study on the influence of exercise and BMI on injuries and illnesses in overweight and obese people showed that jumping right into intensive exercise when your body is simply not ready can be a setup for serious injury. If you carry excess weight, you are at far greater risk for trauma requiring medical attention.[102] The study also showed that the higher your BMI, the higher your risk of sustaining an injury from exercise far more quickly.

WHY MOVEMENT IS STILL IMPORTANT

Having said all that, I absolutely *do* recommend adapting to some type of movement in your day, every day—*eventually* and when you feel ready.

I also like to use the term "movement" rather than exercise. The word "exercise" carries such negative associations for many of us. Feeling overly sweaty, in pain, exhausted, and intimidated in a gym with a lot of fit-looking people is certainly one. Many of my patients have tried exercise programs and either felt absolutely no connection to the activity or have felt bored and irritated.

> **Patient Voice:** BT (female, office manager)
>
> *"I absolutely hate exercise. It hurts, and nothing makes me feel more insecure or worse about my body."*

"Movement" is simpler. Movement carries you throughout your day. Movement can be as small as stretching your arms over your head, eyes closed and breathing deeply. It can be strolling around your living room while on the phone with a friend or walking to the mailbox, chatting to neighbors.

EXERCISE   **MOVEMENT**

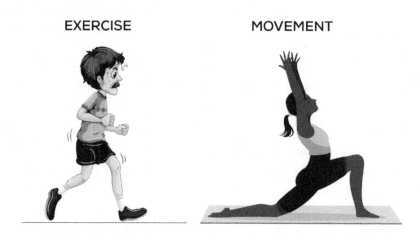

Notice that I said adapting to movement "eventually." This is because if you are out of the habit of movement, or have been really struggling with weight, joint pains, or severely low fatigue, I often find it better to focus on taking off 5–10 lbs. first. Even that small amount of weight loss can boost energy and reduce the likelihood of injury to the joints from overexertion.

Starting a new lifestyle plan with a focus on food first, to get that quick initial loss, can also improve your motivation to start a movement program. Plus, it's a whole lot easier to focus on just *one* thing at a time (like eating changes) and then bring movement in later.

Having said this, it's also true that for some, this strategy can work in reverse.

Sometimes I have patients who are truly struggling to make eating changes right out of the gate. There may be additional factors and stressors such as financial, emotional, or psychological difficulties that pose unique challenges for changing their eating immediately. Or how about the stressors of working full time from home during a pandemic, homeschooling kids, and being unable to shop regularly for healthy food?

Whatever the reason, if the eating changes don't seem to click at first, movement can be a way to implement other health benefits while also improving energy and morale. This is especially true for the postpandemic, sedentary lifestyles that many of us are living. Movement, especially if it can be outdoors, is a wonderful way to get that "buzz" to help lift us emotionally and even spiritually.

HOW TO ADAPT TO MOVEMENT

For those not used to movement, I generally advise something slow and limited at first, such as a 5-to-10-minute walk daily, or 10 minutes of stretching, yoga, tai chi, or chair exercise. There are a ton of free resources on YouTube, or you can join a program such as Launchpadworkouts.com for more personalized guidance.

Other ways to begin movement:

— Take a break at your desk by reaching around to the back of your chair on one side to do a gentle twist, then repeat to the other side.

— Play hide-and-seek with a child.

— Try a fitness video game like Wii, Nike+, or Everybody Dance.

— Grab a friend or family member and head outside to a park for a short walk. Optional: pack a cooler with drinks to relax and enjoy the scenery afterwards.

— Go bowling or to miniature golf.

— Buy a new pet toy and play with your cat or dog (they will love this too!).

— Hop on a bike for a ride. If balance is an issue, three-wheeled trikes are great for all ages.

— Take a stroll around your local mall.

- Visit a local pool or beach (if you're lucky!) and enjoy bobbing and floating in the water.

- The Insight Timer app has a yoga section with a huge variety of free classes streaming daily for all fitness levels—even flat-out beginners who have never tried to stretch before.

The key is that whatever you choose to do, start very slowly, both to avoid injury as well as to make it easier to hit success milestones.

There is no reason to immediately jump into expensive personal training, start running, or join a CrossFit gym (unless you really, really want to!) and risk injury that sours you on the journey. Low-level, consistent movement that becomes part of your routine for life is the goal. Think about it this way: movement is going to become one of the habits that helps you *maintain* your weight loss, rather than getting the weight off in the first place.[103]

• FOOD *for* THOUGHT •
How Muscle Soreness Affects the Scale

Exercising beyond capacity of your muscles will create soreness—that's a fact.

Many patients will also note that their weight drops after exercise but that their overall loss will then temporarily pause, or the scale may even rebound higher than their baseline.

Why?

Answer: the initial sweating after a workout amounts to loss of water weight. However, one to two days postexercise, mild muscle swelling can cause the scale to increase. Muscle swelling is very common with untrained muscles or intensive workouts, so don't despair; once you have healed and recovered, the scale will come right back down where it should be.

Further along the line, movement can be increased as tolerated, and as I always say, *anything* counts, whether it's chasing your kids at the playground, online dance or fitness classes, gym exercise, hiking, or biking. Movement is something you can truly make your own, on your own terms, and in your own time.

Patient Voice: *AH (female, nurse)*

"Exercise now maintains my sanity as well as my weight loss."

CHAPTER TAKEAWAY POINTS

Although movement won't necessarily drive weight loss, it is a critical piece of adjustment that improves our mood and sleep, and lowers stress, while keeping us motivated to continue the journey. And the cardiovascular benefits are outstanding! If you think creatively with the idea of movement, it becomes a lot easier to incorporate into your daily schedule.

SELF-EXPLORATION

Types of movement that appeal to me:

_____

My initial plan and commitment to include movement in my lifestyle plan:

_____

10

TURBO BOOSTERS FOR ADJUSTMENT

"Nothing is impossible. The word itself says, 'I'm Possible!'"
—Attributed to Audrey Hepburn

Losing weight is not always an easy proposition, especially if you are affected by metabolic syndrome or carbohydrate intolerance, as we discussed in earlier chapters.

And the more you've dieted over the years, the harder it can be. I never believe, though, in having to fight your body *too* hard to lose weight. This is why it's important to consider everything possible to optimize conditions for weight loss, which can sometimes include the use of what I call *turbo boosters*.

Using medications or even having weight-loss surgery as a booster is absolutely not a "cop-out," as some might believe. Just like any medical problem requires a comprehensive long-term plan, so does obesity—relying on willpower alone or feeling like you need to "tough it out" by yourself simply flies in the face of everything we know about the biological mechanism of weight gain. The use of turbo boosters is a great way to adjust for common speedbumps that may occur along your journey, like a weight plateau.

TURBO BOOSTER #1: WEIGHT-LOSS PRESCRIPTION MEDICATIONS

Guidelines from the Obesity Medicine Association advise the use of weight-loss medications if patients have not lost 1 lb./week after six months of trying (which equates to 24 lbs. in six months).[104] I personally think this is a bit long to struggle on your own when you are working hard on weight loss and lifestyle change! Because of this, I generally follow the Food and Drug Administration guidelines, which approve weight-loss medications in the following situations, regardless of how long you have tried to change your diet:[105]

- If your BMI is 27 or greater and you have at least one weight-related condition (such as diabetes, hypertension, sleep apnea, or high cholesterol); *or*

- If your BMI is 30 or greater regardless of any weight-related conditions; *and*

- If the medications are to be used in conjunction with lifestyle modifications—in other words, the medications are part of an adjustment to a lifestyle plan that you are already in the process of adapting to.

Medications cannot be used by women who are pregnant or breastfeeding, and for anyone with a history of eating disorders or substance abuse, I recommend their use with caution.

In my practice, I feel medications can be very helpful if patients have a long history of difficulty with weight loss, have plateaued, or are hitting any other speedbumps. However, I also feel it makes sense to optimize any and all conditions first. The aim of using medications is to grease the wheels, so to speak, so there isn't much sense in throwing on weight-loss pills and expecting a miracle unless I have first analyzed a patient's entire situation inside and out. There *is no* magic pill, and weight-loss medications will produce varying degrees of weight loss and at variable rates for different people.

FACTORS TO CONSIDER WITH ANY WEIGHT-LOSS MEDICATION

– Diet and lifestyle changes should be in place first or at least be used in conjunction with medication use. This is based on research data demonstrating the effectiveness of weight-loss medications—all of which were studied *along with* diet and lifestyle, not separate from diet and lifestyle. The effects of drugs without lifestyle change are modest at best[106] and, in my opinion, not worth the risk of side effects, drug interactions, or potential intolerances that can occur. I have even seen some patients gain weight while taking them.

– Even though, for many patients, the risk of carrying excess weight outweighs the risk of a reaction or side effect with a drug, medication always carries that potential risk, which I like to make sure patients understand.

– The effects of weight-loss medications are generally temporary. This is because no matter what hunger pathway can be blocked with a drug, the body will eventually find a way around it. As mentioned earlier, the regulation of weight is highly complex! So, if you do take weight-loss medication, expect the peak effect within the first one to three months. After that time, you may notice less of an impact on your hunger and weight-loss trajectory.

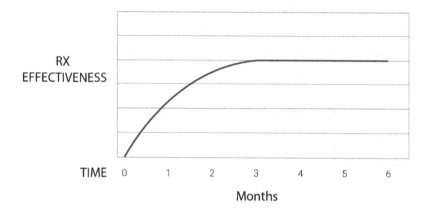

- Consider using medications in conjunction with other turbo boosters such as bariatric surgery. Research carried out at Harvard Medical School has shown that after bariatric surgery, starting patients on weight-loss medications once a weight plateau is reached can help them achieve an additional 7.6% weight loss beyond what bariatric surgery alone can offer.[107]

- Before any weight-loss medication is prescribed, you should work with your doctor to eliminate or reduce doses wherever possible of any existing medications that might be causing weight gain or impeding weight loss (refer to Chapter 4 for more on what these are). There isn't much sense in taking medication if its effects are only going to be negated by other drugs in your body.

CURRENT FDA-APPROVED WEIGHT-LOSS MEDICATIONS[108]

1. The phenylethylamine class of medications, including phentermine, diethylpropion, and phendimetrazine (brand names Adipex, Fastin, Lomaira, Bontril, Tenuate)

Phenylethylamines are stimulant medications that speed up the metabolism and reduce appetite by acting on areas of the brain that control these functions. They are the oldest class of weight-loss drugs, having first been launched in the 1940s and 1950s in the USA. Despite bad publicity surrounding the use of a phenylethylamine drug called fenfluramine-phentermine (fen-phen), which caused serious cardiac side effects, the phenylethylamines currently available are generally a safe class of drugs. Fewer than 1% of people who use them have side effects (which can include palpitations, fast heart rate, elevated blood pressure, headache, dry mouth, dizziness, or kidney stones). These drugs, however, are not for use by anyone who has advanced cardiac disease or uncontrolled blood pressure.

2. Phentermine and topiramate (brand name Qsymia).

This drug is a combination of phentermine and topiramate, a drug which, interestingly, is FDA-approved for seizures but is frequently used by physicians "off-label" for migraines, anxiety, and weight control on its own, as weight loss is frequently noted as one of its side effects. The mechanism by which topiramate causes weight loss is unknown, but aside from its own effects, it seems to boost the power of phentermine when they are taken together. The adverse effects and cautions are similar to those above for phentermine alone.

3. Liraglutide (brand name Saxenda)

The newer drug liraglutide is by far my favorite FDA-approved weight-loss medication. The mechanism by which it controls appetite and weight is almost a biochemical bariatric surgery, if you will: liraglutide gives patients a sense of fullness with very little food intake by slowing the emptying of the gut as well as by transmitting hormonal signals to the brain signaling fullness. It works especially well with low-carb eating and has a powerful impact. Liraglutide is also marketed as a diabetes drug (brand name Victoza) so it's an excellent choice for those with type 2 diabetes or prediabetes. The main side effect of liraglutide is nausea, which occurs in 10%–20% of users, however the nausea tends to get better after the first two weeks. Less frequently reported side effects are constipation, upset stomach, and headache. It can't be used in those who have had pancreatitis or a certain type of rare thyroid cancer, but these are fairly unusual conditions. So, what's the downside of liraglutide? First: it's an injection, not a capsule, although having used it myself I find the injection pen needle to be far less painful than pricking my finger to check blood sugar. And second: cost. Many insurance companies are still balking at covering the $1,000+/month bill for its use. To me, this is a terrible shame, given that the health costs of obesity annually are far greater than this. I'm hopeful that the tide will change as more and more patients show benefits with this drug.

4. Bupropion and Naltrexone (Brand name Contrave)

Contrave combines the antidepressant bupropion with naltrexone, a drug that acts on the brain to powerfully reduce cravings. Bupropion is interesting in that it is biochemically similar to a phenylethylamine medication, even though it behaves differently. Contrave is a medication with more drug interactions and a higher profile of side effects, including elevated blood pressure, dizziness, nausea, constipation, dry mouth, and liver abnormalities, which can occur in 10% of patients. Cost is also an issue with this medication, as no generic is available as of the time of writing.

5. Orlistat (Brand name Xenical; also available over the counter as Alli)

Orlistat blocks enzymes in the gut that digest fat. Unlike other FDA-approved weight-loss medications, only orlistat is available (at a lower strength) without a prescription over the counter. I have to say that of all the medications above, orlistat is probably my least favorite. Most patients find the side effects pretty intolerable, and the achieved weight loss is *very* minimal (studies show 2–3 lbs. at about one year). Plus, given orlistat's mechanism (blocking fat absorption, causing the fat you eat to be excreted in stool), it is generally ill-advised on a low-carb eating plan where plenty of healthy fat is consumed—what's the point?

6. Cellulose and citric acid (Brand name Plenity—FDA-approved but not yet widely available at the time of writing)

   Plenity is an entirely different type of medication, which comes in capsule form. When swallowed, the capsule releases thousands of particles into the stomach that rapidly absorb water and expand, creating a feeling of fullness without any caloric value. Plenity is fairly safe except for those with certain stomach conditions, and I expect wide release of this medication soon.

I mentioned above that medications can be prescribed "off-label." This means that although they are not technically FDA-approved for the purpose of weight loss, they are perfectly legal for doctors to prescribe. One example of this is the drug semaglutide, which works in a similar way to liraglutide. Although only FDA-approved to treat type 2 diabetes and not for obesity, semaglutide's weight-loss power for individuals without diabetes was demonstrated in a large trial published in February 2021 in the *New England Journal of Medicine*.

When using medications off-label, it's important for you and your doctor to be even more alert to any potential side effects or drug interactions that may occur. When I prescribe off-label, I try to match the medication's use with any other conditions my patient has that the medication might help. For example, if you have a history of migraines and are trying to lose weight, we might give topiramate a try, which is used as migraine-preventive medication.

> **Patient Voice:** GM (female, attorney)
>
> *"I realize that the medication can't do it all and it won't work forever. But by taking 'the edge' off my hunger, it helps me feel so much more in control of what I eat."*

• FOOD *for* THOUGHT •
"Off-label" medications that can assist with weight loss[109]

Topiramate (brand name Topamax)

Zonisamide

Bupropion (brand name Wellbutrin)

Metformin

Semaglutide (brand names Ozempic and Rybelsus)

Liraglutide (brand name Victoza)

Here are some drugs that I do *not* recommend for use as weight-loss medication.

1. SGLT-2 (Sodium glucose cotransporter 2) inhibitor drugs

    These diabetes medications that typically end in "-gliflozin" have the trade names Jardiance, Farxiga, Invokana, and Steglatro. They are associated with a modest 3% weight loss in research studies,[110] however in conjunction with a low-carb diet, they can result in a very serious side effect called euglycemic ketoacidosis, meaning that dangerous levels of acids build up in the blood without elevating the blood sugar levels, making it a difficult condition to detect.[111] This condition can even be fatal if not recognized and treated promptly. Not worth the risk, in my opinion.

2. The use of thyroid hormone specifically for weight loss

    I occasionally encounter patients to whom certain practitioners have recommended thyroid hormone supplements for weight loss. These should be avoided at all costs, as excess thyroid supplementation carries the risk of causing abnormal heart rhythms, bone density loss, and anxiety, among other concerns.[112] It doesn't even generally result in weight loss. To me, the extent to which the thyroid influences weight is actually smaller than many people realize.[113] It can account for several pounds, but not 50. Large weight gains are not typical with hypothyroid but *are* very typical of metabolic syndrome. Don't get me wrong—if you have been diagnosed with low thyroid hormone levels, you absolutely need to be treated for this. But this treatment is for establishing thyroid hormone balance in the body, *not* for excess weight specifically. If a patient is taking such a supplement, I generally advise that they stop immediately.

TURBO BOOSTER #2: WEIGHT-LOSS SURGERY

It may sound drastic, but weight-loss surgery can be a valid option to consider. For some people, their obesity persists despite their best attempts at lifestyle changes. In some cases, someone may reach a plateau that even medications do not help with. This can lead to an incredible amount of frustration, and I find patients get fed up and lose heart with maintaining healthy lifestyle habits.

In particular, if your obesity is severe (BMI >40), your chances of achieving and maintaining what is defined as a normal BMI is less than 1%.[114] But it's not all about the scale, either. Weight-loss surgery has been shown to effectively treat weight-associated diseases like type 2 diabetes, sleep apnea, hypertension, high cholesterol, arthritis, and acid reflux. Surgery also reduces the risk of death from these issues plus the risk of many common cancers by over 40%.[115] That's why surgery should at least be a consideration if you qualify.

Weight-loss surgery works by both restricting the amount of food that you eat and by changing some of the hunger hormone signaling in the gut, making it easier to lose weight. Approximately 90% of patients lose 50% of their excess body weight after bariatric surgery and keep the weight off long-term.[116] But don't stop reading the rest of this book just yet: without a long-term commitment to changing your diet and lifestyle, surgery won't work well on its own.

But is it safe? Extensive studies carried out by the American Society for Bariatric and Metabolic Surgery (ASMBS) have found that the risk of death from any cause ends up being far lower for patients undergoing weight-loss surgery than for those who have severe obesity and never have surgery. From the ASMBS website:

> *"Decades ago, weight loss surgery was seen as high risk and the rewards were seen as mostly cosmetic. This is completely incorrect. The risk of death due to surgery is very low in the first year after surgery, about the same as gallbladder surgery or knee replacement surgery. Surgery for weight loss lowers the risk of death related to many diseases including heart disease (40% lower), diabetes (92% lower), and cancer (60% lower).... Comparing the risks of surgery to the benefits of surgery makes the decision for surgery much easier to make."*[117]

Criteria on selecting surgical candidates for weight-loss surgery are also in flux. Current National Institute of Health criteria are as follows:

- BMI >40 (regardless of health conditions)
- BMI >35 with one serious, excess weight-related medical comorbidity

And, in some cases, you may be approved for weight-loss surgery at an even lower BMI if you have type 2 diabetes that has not been well controlled with medication.

If you choose the surgical route, it is critical that surgery be performed by a board-certified surgeon with specialized experience or training in bariatric and metabolic surgery and at a center that has a multidisciplinary team of experts. If the hospital even has a postbariatric surgery recovery unit, all the better. The team of experts may include a registered dietitian, an exercise physiologist or physical therapist to aid in postoperative movement, and a clinical psychologist with bariatric expertise.

In addition, some insurance companies require that the surgery be performed at a facility that meets the ASMBS-approved quality standards, which are outlined by an organization called The Metabolic and Bariatric Surgery Accreditation and Quality Improvement Program, or MBSAQIP.[118] The MBSAQIP-approved facilities must meet certain regulations and requirements for the care of bariatric patients, including both inpatient procedures on admission and provisions for outpatient long-term follow-up, which is key to helping patients achieve success.

TYPES OF WEIGHT-LOSS SURGERY

It's beyond the scope of this book to talk extensively about the many types of procedures, but here I list the types of surgeries most typically discussed with patients with some basic information about each one.[119]

1. Laparoscopic Roux-en-Y gastric bypass. This procedure works by both restricting the amount of food that can be taken into the stomach and bypassing the first portion of the intestine where the bulk of calories is absorbed into the body.

2. Vertical sleeve gastrectomy. The "sleeve," as it is popularly known, is a purely restrictive procedure that reduces the stomach size—you end up with a banana-shaped stomach rather than a large sac. Therefore, it is more difficult to eat large portions.

3. Laparoscopic gastric banding. The "band" is a device that encircles the top portion of the stomach, also restricting the amount of food that can be eaten. This is the only surgery that is fully reversible. However, it's important to know that in some cases surgery may be required to remove the band if it slips or erodes the stomach and causes some damage as a result.

4.   Duodenal switch. This is similar to a gastric bypass, but more of the intestine is bypassed.

5.   Intragastric balloon (not really a surgery, as no part of your anatomy is altered in any way.) The balloon is inserted into the stomach then inflated, left in place for a defined period of time, and then removed.

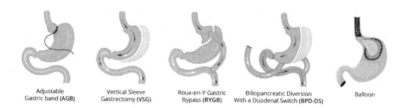

| Adjustable Gastric band (AGB) | Vertical Sleeve Gastrectomy (VSG) | Roux-en-Y Gastric Bypass (RYGB) | Biliopancreatic Diversion With a Duodenal Switch (BPD-DS) | Balloon |

Procedures (1) and (2) are by far the most commonly performed bariatric surgeries nowadays, with the sleeve growing enormously in popularity as it is a simpler surgery to perform and can be done on a wider range of patients. Surgeons have been shying away from (3), the band, as longer-term data are showing inconsistent weight loss plus higher complication risks that often necessitate band removal. Procedure (4), the switch, is rarely performed, having been replaced largely by the gastric bypass as there are far fewer long-term side effects.[120] I fully expect to see newer, less invasive procedures like the balloon (5) growing in popularity over the next five years, even though we don't yet have extensive long-term data on its effectiveness like true bariatric surgery. A discussion with your surgeon can help you to decide which is the best procedure for your needs and particular medical concerns.

Bear in mind, though, that surgery is still surgery, and complications can occur. One long-term issue from surgery is that vitamins are not well absorbed afterwards, so patients must commit to taking daily vitamins for life. But that's better than insulin shots for life, right?

It's also critical to understand that surgery is not a cure-all but rather is just one way to adjust and turbo boost; a lifelong, low-carb eating plan is still critical for success. I also feel low-carb eating fits in quite well with bariatric surgery patients because

— most individuals who gain enough weight to require surgery have metabolic syndrome at baseline and

— side effects of bariatric surgery, which can include nausea and diarrhea, are greatly reduced by eliminating sugars and simple starches, which would happen on a low-carb eating plan.

Some of my patients wonder if having bariatric surgery means that they have failed with their diet in some way—and the answer to this is unequivocally *no*. Remember in Chapter 3 how we discussed the high weight set point that develops after we gain weight? Helping you to push past the set point is one of the key advantages that bariatric surgery can give you. Medications can do this too, but they don't have nearly the same effectiveness.

Key questions to ask yourself if you are considering bariatric surgery:

1. Do I meet FDA criteria for surgery?
2. Which procedure interests me?
3. Am I geographically close to (or can I travel to) a bariatric center of excellence, as defined by the ASMBS and MBSAQIP? Living close to the center makes having a successful procedure that much more likely. And remember, having success means not just getting through surgery and the recovery period— it also includes ongoing follow-up and care for at least five years. ASMBS member surgeons in the US can be found here: https://asmbs.org/patients/find-a-provider.

TURBO BOOSTER #3: NONPRESCRIPTION SUPPLEMENTS

Do a Google search of "weight-loss supplements," and you'll come up with a myriad of sites selling all sorts of nonprescription supplement pills.

When you've been struggling with weight for a long time, it makes sense to try whatever it takes, right?

It's a huge industry; consumers spend $32 billion a year on over-the-counter supplements that claim to treat all kinds of problems, including excess weight.[121] Regardless of whether they work, the first thing anyone needs to know is whether a supplement is safe or whether it can cause harm. This is not always an easy question to answer because there is little regulation of the industry as a whole. Unlike pharmaceutical drugs, which must prove to the FDA that they are both safe and effective, supplements are presumed to be safe and effective unless they are proven otherwise. To me, this is quite scary!

The biggest area of concern for dietary supplements is the issue of contamination—sometimes with unrelated chemicals, but other times with actual medications that are no longer available. This is particularly rampant in the weight-loss supplements category.[122]

For example, sibutramine, which was pulled off the market in 2010 due to increased risk of cardiac events and strokes,[123] is now showing up as an ingredient in some of these supplements.

There are also reports of supplements containing the prescription drug lorcaserin that you can buy on the Internet. What makes this especially worrying is that lorcaserin was actually taken off the market in 2020 as it was found to increase the risk of several types of cancers. It is no longer available by prescription.[124]

So, while you might well experience a beneficial effect from a supplement, because these are nonregulated products you may be opening yourself up to a lot of adverse effects. Additionally, your physician may not even know that you have been exposed to that pharmaceutical compound. Even if you take a supplement brand that you discover is pure and safe, some supplements can affect the liver and kidneys just like other medications can, so I would always strongly advise monitoring.

There are other concerns related to drug interactions. An example might be a patient taking a blood thinner who also decides to take ginkgo biloba. The interaction between a certain blood pressure medication and ginkgo biloba can result in increased blood pressure, which can dramatically increase risk for bleeding—definitely not what we want to see. For all these reasons, the Obesity Medicine Association does not recommend that doctors encourage patients to use supplements for weight loss.[125]

• FOOD *for* THOUGHT •

How Publication Bias Makes Supplements Seem More Effective Than They Are:[126]

— The disproportionate number of positive results compared to negative results compromises the objectivity of research reviews and what are known as "meta-analyses"—analyses of large groups of studies that are often used to interpret the effectiveness of studies in aggregate.

— Negative or insignificant study results on supplements are rarely promoted and are less likely to be submitted to scientific journals for publication. As a result, all we end up hearing about in the media are positive results, which on the whole, are generally due to very small and poorly done studies.

Bottom line on supplements: proceed at your own risk (both health-wise and the risk to your wallet!). If you do decide to try one, a good resource for both doctors and patients regarding supplements is the US Pharmacopeia.[127] Data on safety, purity, and interaction potential for USP-certified supplements are available on the site. Be sure to check the supplements you are taking here. If what you are taking is not USP-certified, there may be cause for concern. Another good site to investigate is The Natural Medicines Database.[128]

Of the available supplements for weight loss on the market, there are very limited data on their effectiveness in clinical trials. Here are a few that are probably among the safest:

1. Fiber capsules

    It's always best to get fiber from the diet via adequate green leafy veg-etable intake, but extra fiber may be beneficial in certain situations, for example, if you suffer from constipation despite adequate dietary fiber from other sources. One of the most common ingredients in fiber capsules is psyllium, which comes from plant husks (this is also the main ingredient in the product Metamucil). Another type of prebiotic fiber is inulin. Fiber slows digestion and can make you feel more full, causing you to eat a little less and potentially helping to prevent abdominal weight gain.[129] But beware: too much fiber can cause bloating, heartburn, gas, or even an intestinal blockage. Always drink at least 8–10 oz of water with each capsule to prevent any problems. Fiber capsules may also interfere with the absorption of some commonly used medications for depression, diabetes, high cholesterol, thyroid disorders, heart problems, and seizures, so it's best to take the capsules one to two hours apart from any medica-tions that treat these conditions. In general, fiber capsules are fairly inexpensive compared with other supplements.

2. Ketone supplements

    If you are eating a low-carb diet, you have probably heard about taking supplemental ketones in the forms of powders, bars, or drinks to help reduce hunger and speed weight loss. It is believed that ke-tones produced by the body have an anti-hunger effect, but the jury is still out on whether taking extra ketones has any effect on weight loss.[130] Ketone supplements are generally considered safe, but we don't know what short- or long-term effects these supplements could have on the body. No good studies exist yet on potential side effects or interactions with commonly used medications.

3. Green tea

   The use of green tea for health benefits began in China thousands of years ago.[131] It is considered healthy as a beverage due to high concentrations of catechins, polyphenols, and epigallocatechin gallate, which act as antioxidants in the body. Research on weight-loss effect has been mixed with some studies showing a possible effect, others more minimal.[132] Most studies have been done with very small sample sizes, too, so it's difficult to generalize to larger groups of people. It's also not clear how much the caffeine content in the tea plays a role, as caffeine, in itself, is a stimulant. However, on the whole, studies don't show a great appetite-suppression effect.[133] There are concerns with green tea: those with hypertension, heart arrhythmias or heart disease in general, anxiety, or insomnia could find these conditions worsen.

4. Lovidia

   This is a supplement pill composed of food ingredients that are "generally recognized as safe" including stevia leaf, berberine, and natural flavorings in a slow-release capsule. Small, very preliminary research sponsored by the manufacturer shows that individuals can have a modest decrease in weight, hunger, blood sugars, and cholesterol when taking Lovidia compared to a pill without the ingredient in it.[134] Caveats: not all consumers experience the Lovidia effect—there seem to be responders and nonresponders, and it's impossible to predict who will respond without just trying it. There are no known side effects or medication interactions, and the company at the time of writing was offering a money-back guarantee. Disclaimer: I am an advisor to this company.

5. Gamma-linolenic acid (GLA)

   GLA is an activated form of omega-6 fatty acids. Fatty acids are critical for many body functions including cell nourishment, decreased inflammation, hormonal balance, and skin nourishment.[135] GLA is something breast-fed infants obtain from their mothers' milk. Formula-fed infants and older children and adults don't get a large supply of these activated fatty acids through diet. Theoretically, GLA can stimulate fat burning by activating prostaglandins. Reliable data are lacking, but GLA is being actively studied for its role in weight loss. Dietary sources of GLA include evening primrose oil or borage seed oil, both of which are felt to be generally safe.

Before taking any supplements, remember that general Internet searches and social media chat rooms are *never* the best source of information. Always speak to your physician first.

Regardless of how you turbo boost your weight loss, I can't emphasize enough that healthy lifestyle habits are the best medicine. Turbo boosters grease the wheels of weight loss, but they don't drive the train! It's far too easy for someone to take a pill, or have a surgery, and lose all the weight they want but then regain it all (and more) without a long-term plan in place. Changing your eating and your mindset around food is 100% essential—no pill, supplement, or surgical procedure can take its place!

CHAPTER TAKEAWAY POINTS

Turbo boosters for weight loss can be helpful, including FDA-approved and off-label medications for weight loss as well as bariatric surgery. The evidence for over-the-counter supplement use is weak at best. Working with an experienced physician to incorporate a turbo booster for weight loss is essential.

11

ADAPTING AND ADJUSTING FOR LIFE

"Progress is more important than perfection."
—*Simon Sinek, best-selling author and speaker*

You've achieved the goal you have created for yourself and have been striving toward—congratulations! It won't have been easy all the way along, but I hope you feel it has been worth it.

As you get closer to a health goal or weight that you feel comfortable maintaining, you may have experienced some of the following:

First—initial euphoria when you realize that "it's working"—you are actually losing weight despite prior struggles.

This is, of course, incredibly exciting and rewarding and can help shape your motivation to continue for life. However, it's important to remember that just like any emotion, motivation can wax and wane over time. This is not a reason to give up on your goals. Acknowledge that motivation may be low at times. Motivation increases or decreases naturally, and certainly as a result of what else is going on in your life. For example, it's tough to feel motivated when you are in the midst of a severe personal crisis or struggling financially. Know that this is perfectly okay—don't beat yourself up or punish yourself for feeling less energetic about your health goals from time to time. Even just recognizing and telling yourself something as simple as, "I notice my motivation is a bit lower right now," can help you coast through the period without being derailed. And, remembering your *why* (Chapter 2) is critical for boosting motivation, now and forever!

• FOOD *for* THOUGHT •
Remembering Your *Why* (patient voices)

"I never want to have to take blood pressure medication again."

"Hearing that my kidneys are starting to fail is terrifying."

"I don't want my kids to go through what I've had to with my health issues."

"I never want to have to do those insulin shots like my dad did before he died."

"I want to feel beautiful and sexy for once in my life."

"I never want to be called names because of my size by anyone again."

"I want to run and play with my grandkids without my knees acting up."

"I don't want to feel controlled by food anymore."

What's *yours?*

Second—recognition from others that you look and *are* different. You may be enjoying the rewarding feeling of looser clothes. Your doctor may be congratulating you on improvements in medical problems as well. However, for those who have lost large amounts of weight, the changes in body shape might, in reality, be upsetting. Why would this be?

— You may experience pushback from those around you, be they friends, family, or coworkers as you continue to work on the healthy habits that will help you maintain. Commonly heard by my patients are the following:

> "You look good—why are you so worried? Just have a dough-nut with me," or "a small bowl of fried noodles won't hurt you."

> "You are *way* too skinny now."

> "Aren't you worried that if you keep losing weight you will have all that hanging skin?"

> If this is the case for you, refer back to the "Speedbumps and Roadblocks" chapter on social eating for handy responses and quotes. In some cases, such as with closer family and friends, a frank discussion to address the issue may be necessary, which is not always easy or comfortable to do. Remember that you are only accountable to yourself, and in the end, only you have to live with the health problems and emotional pain that can come with feel-ing unhealthy. You don't owe anyone anything!

— You may even experience guilt at having put your health and per-sonal needs first. For example, one of my patients expressed guilt at having to spend money to buy new clothes at a time during the pandemic when her family was struggling financially. Many of us pride ourselves on being "givers"—always there to care for children, elders, friends, or coworkers—and as a result we put our health and our bodies last on the list of things to care for. Over time, we become less healthy and more sick because of this mindset, and then who does this serve? You can't give to others without giving to yourself first, so sweep away that guilt!

— For others, there is even shame or the feeling that you are undeserv-ing of your successes. You may even feel like you have lost part of yourself or that you are disappearing. If you have always identified as being larger, there may be an uncomfortable sense that part of your identity is now gone. Re-examining your motives can be helpful: Who was the weight loss for again? Do you feel responsible for the feelings of others? What was your *why*?

If you are experiencing these types of difficulties, or if you have a history of trauma that has influenced your eating, this is where skilled psychotherapy can make a big difference. The right emotional support can keep you on track to make ongoing adjustments, which are needed to maintain your weight loss. It can also help you with mental clarity as you continue to adapt and adjust to maintain health for life.

Third—acceptance of where you are. This may be the most powerful accomplishment of all! Perhaps you ended up revising the goal of being your high-school weight to something more modest. Maybe lowering doses of medications or having less joint pain while walking feels so wonderful that the number on the scale feels much less pertinent. Maybe you have cultivated more body positivity and have achieved more mental clarity with your changes. These are all fantastic and you may find you've gained a lot of satisfaction from these accomplishments. Remember that no matter our weight, genetics are a powerful shaper of our shapes, so it's not realistic for all of us to look like fitness models or buff bodybuilders or to push ourselves to the extent that we create deep unhappiness for ourselves. As we've discussed in prior chapters, even a 5%–10% weight loss has profound health benefits. Accepting and celebrating where you are is therefore a huge achievement in itself!

Many of my patients express worry that in "maintenance," they will regain weight when they "go off the diet." You can avoid these pitfalls by following these pillars of maintenance or adjustments for life.

1. Continue to fuel up primarily with proteins/greens/fats, the body's essential macronutrients. This will also help control hunger and cravings. Keep veggies dark, green, and low carb as much as possible.

   A common question I am asked is, "How do I know how many carbs I can eat to maintain my weight?" This is critical and is different for each individual. I like to call this one's "carb-tolerance limit." Everyone's limit is different, and if you've been on the weight-loss journey for some time, you probably now have a better idea of how much you can safely eat. But as your body changes, the carb-tolerance limit will likely also change. It may decrease as your body continues to fight back against weight loss. Hopefully, if you've started to incorporate movement, it has at least stabilized or even increased—remember that when we build muscle, we become more insulin-sensitive, meaning we can better tolerate higher amounts of carbohydrates in the diet.

   Some people prefer to eat extremely low carb as a lifelong plan, with occasional "splurge days" as a weight maintenance tool. This is perfectly valid if it works for you. Others use ongoing intermittent fasting as part of their toolbox to maintain. There is no one right way.

• FOOD *for* THOUGHT •
How to Find Your Own Carb-Tolerance Limit

Try adding in one serving of extras (from the list in Chapter 4) daily for two weeks. At the end of two weeks, weigh yourself. If the scale is the same, that's great. It means that you are still eating under your carb-tolerance limit.

Repeat as often as you like. If you notice the scale increasing two weeks after adding in an extra, you may need to reevaluate or make other adjustments to continue to eat your desired extra.

2. Practice *hara hachi bu*, eating until you are only 80% full.[136] This cultural practice from Japan can increase mindfulness and is critical to maintaining your weight. Eat slowly, pausing between each bite. Concentrate on noticing the feeling of food not only in your mouth but also as you swallow and as food gradually begins to fill your stomach. The 80% goal helps avoid overstuffing and keeps you feeling in control of your eating (rather than it being the other way around).

3. Use fallback foods to navigate difficult situations. What do I mean by this? Fallback foods are those you can "fall back on" as go-tos when you are either attending a gathering or eating out where there may not be the healthiest choices available. Always look to raw veggies or salad and protein as fallback foods, which should generally be available. And never go to any event feeling hungry.

4. Watch grazing. Especially during the COVID-19 pandemic, with more of us at home and feeling bored and irritable a lot of the time, it's easy to turn to the fridge or pantry for a nibble here and there. These haphazard eating patterns are dangerous, as they cause insulin levels to stay elevated constantly, reinforcing fat stores and increasing inflammation in the body. Constant snacking also disturbs your body's hunger and satiety signals. Keep eating times structured to three times a day wherever possible, with no more than one snack per day. If you find yourself with more hunger and cravings, check in with your food choices. Are you still sticking to proteins/greens/fats for the most part? Eating the right foods will minimize the desire to graze, while higher amounts of extras will lead to more cravings. Take inventory of what's in your pantry and remove those foods that are especially tempting to you. Also, it can be helpful to check in with your feelings when you are tempted to graze—are you bored, anxious, tired, or stressed? Practice awareness of these emotions and try to find ways to soothe them. A five-minute walk outside the house and away from your screen can help you reset.

5. Consider intermittent fasting (discussed earlier) as a way to help your body keep adjusting. IF is a great way to allow insulin levels to fall, activating your body's fat-burning machinery in a powerful way.

6. Prioritize your flowing needs and your own emotional well-being. Keep your needs for rest, self-care, sleep, and recharge time a high priority. This may require schedule changes, a pay cut, a change in relationship dynamics, or even a new job for some. You can do anything, but you can't do everything.

7. Prioritize your general health. Make sure you get regular check-ups from your primary physician and attend all routine health screenings (mammograms, colonoscopies, routine blood work, and vaccinations as recommended).

8. Be active. Many of you will likely have started some type of movement, even if it's just 10 minutes of walking per day. The more the better at this point. As discussed in Chapter 7, though, the idea is not to burn calories but to improve your overall fitness level and heart health, while preserving muscle tone and boosting motivation levels. The more active you are, the more sensitive your muscles will be to insulin's effects, keeping metabolic syndrome in check.

• FOOD *for* THOUGHT •
Making Movement Stick

– Schedule regular movement time in your calendar. Sign up for Zoom fitness classes and add them to your agenda for reinforcement. Aim to move daily, even if in small amounts.

– Find a fitness buddy, either online or in person, for accountability.

– Keep it simple: a quick daily walk is easy to implement, is free, and doesn't require special equipment.

- Experiment to find something you enjoy. It could be Zumba, swimming, yoga, barre method, dancing, weights, or the popular Swedish exercise "plogging" (picking up trash as you walk your neighborhood— it does a good deed in the community *and* gets a variety of movement in including walking, squatting, twisting and stretching!)[137]

9. Consider weighing yourself regularly. I'm not a huge fan of daily weighing for everyone, as it can sometimes make you feel neurotic. Many of us have a difficult relationship with our scales and feel they have never been kind to us. If this is the case, it may take time to see the scale as simply a tool and not a cruel, judgmental foe. We never want the tone of your day to be dictated by the number on the scale, and it's common for those numbers to fluctuate daily by as much as two to four pounds. Having said that, we also don't want to lose touch with reality if our weight is starting to climb again. Weight gain is a natural process for our body, and it's quite easy to gain half a pound monthly if we are not mindful. In a year this would equate to six pounds, which is still not a lot, however year over year all weight lost would eventually be regained. So, weighing in once or twice a week should be plenty to reinforce self-monitoring and personal responsibility. Be consistent in your weigh-in routine: do so at a similar time of the day, wear the same clothes (or weigh naked) to get as accurate a reading as possible.

• FOOD *for* THOUGHT •
What to Do If the Scale Scares You?

- Other self-monitoring ideas to consider:
- Take a weekly selfie.

- Measure your waist with a tape measure once a week. Increased waist circumference correlates with the risk of metabolic disease. Lowest risk for biological females: <35", males <40".

- Reduce weigh-ins to once a month.

10. Hydrate, hydrate, hydrate! Aim for 80–100 oz or 2 L of free fluids daily. Good hydration gives you energy and can help reduce between-meal hunger, plus it's essential if you are doing any kind of intermittent fasting to avoid dehydration symptoms like lightheadedness or dizziness. I have to admit, I'm not the best plain water drinker in the world, but I find that drinking sparkling water or flavoring my water with a slice of lemon or lime works wonders. You can also try sugar-free Branched Chain Amino Acid drinks or other flavorings—whatever you enjoy.

11. Don't let your eating slips turn into slides. If you feel your eating patterns starting to slide off into older unhealthy habits, seek help immediately. For example, it's normal to indulge during the holidays or at a special event. But if you find yourself habitually returning to old ways, it's time to check in *before* there is significant weight gain. Look to your physician, a registered low-carb-friendly dietitian, or a group for support. Remember, no one is invincible, including you! I've said before and continue to say that weight gain is entirely natural for the body. And, crucially, the monitoring of the chronic disease of metabolic syndrome doesn't end after weight loss—it requires a lifetime of vigilance and support.

A few final summary points as we close.

Throughout this book, you've heard me speak of a wide variety of approaches and techniques to improve and maintain your metabolic health, from mindset shifts, to eating changes, to movement, medications, and even weight-loss surgery.

I'd like to reiterate a point from Chapter 1 as you digest the "buffet" of all the options and suggestions I've proposed here. And that is, given that no two people are alike, the decision on how you'll continue adapting and adjusting for life is ultimately up to you! There are many pieces of your puzzle to fit together, and the shape of the finished project will vary widely from person to person.

Last but not least, remember:

No matter where you are in life, how old you are, how sick you are, or how badly off you feel, it's always possible to stand up, dust yourself off, dry your tears, and move forward into the light of better health.

We've got this!

12

RESOURCES

Excellent and reputable websites for more information on low-carb lifestyles

Lowcarbusa.org

Virtahealth.com

Dietdoctor.com

Lowcarbcardiologist.com

Thefastingmethod.com

Metabolicpractitioners.org

TedEytan.com

Ketogenic.com

Obesity as a disease resources

Obesity.org

Obesitymedicine.org

Obesityaction.org

Recipe websites (including recipes for items mentioned in earlier chapters)

Lowcarbyum.com

Gnom-Gnom.com

Alldayidreamaboutfood.com

Jenniferbanz.com

Defyfoods.com

Counseling Resources

Plushcare.com/profile/book/therapy/

Psychologytoday.com

Betterhelp.com

Dranitajohnston.com

Apps

Carbmanager.com

Myfitnesspal.com

Eat.selectivor.com

Insighttimer.com

Ketodietapp.com

Movement resources

Launchpadworkouts.com

Mypacer.com

Doyogawithme.com

Healthline.com/nutrition/how-to-start-exercising

Bariatric surgery information

American Society for Metabolic and Bariatric Surgery's patient information

Asmbs.org/patients

American College of Surgeons patient information

Facs.org/quality-programs/mbsaqip

ENDNOTES

1   Keck School of Medicine of USC. "3 Public Global Public Health Threats."
    February 26, 2020. https://mphdegree.usc.edu/blog/3-global-public-health-threats/.

2   Mayo Clinic. "Metabolic Syndrome." Last modified March 14, 2019. https://www.
    mayoclinic.org/diseases-conditions/metabolic-syndrome/symptoms-causes/syc-
    20351916#:~:text=Metabolic%20syndrome%20is%20a%20cluster,abnormal%20
    cholesterol%20or%20triglyceride%20levels. Accessed February 24, 2021.

3   Araújo, Joana, Jianwen Cai, and June Stevens. "Prevalence of Optimal Metabolic
    Health in American Adults: National Health and Nutrition Examination Survey
    2009-2016." *Metabolic Syndrome and Related Disorders* 17, no. 1 (February 8,
    2019): 46–52. https://doi.org/10.1089/met.2018.0105.

4   Rosenweig, James L., George L Bakris, Lars F Berglund, Marie-France Hivert,
    Edward S Horton, Rita R Kalyani, M Hassan Murad, and Bruno L Vergès.
    "Primary Prevention of ASCVD And T2DM in Patients at Metabolic Risk: An
    Endocrine Society Clinical Practice Guideline." *Journal of Clinical Endocrinology
    and Metabolism* 104, no. 9 (July 31, 2019): 3939–85. https://doi.org/10.1210/
    jc.2019-01338.

5   Jane E. Brody. "The Dangers of Belly Fat." *New York Times*, June 11, 2018. https://
    www.nytimes.com/2018/06/11/well/live/belly-fat-health-visceral-fat-waist-cancer.
    html.

6   Cummings, Matthew J., Matthew R. Baldwin, Darryl Abrams, Samuel D.
    Jacobson, Benjamin J. Meyer, Elizabeth M. Balough, Justin G. Aaron, et al.
    "Epidemiology, Clinical Course, and Outcomes of Critically Ill Adults with
    COVID-19 in New York City: A Prospective Cohort Study." *Lancet* 395, no. 10239
    (June 6, 2020): 1763–70. https://doi.org/10.1016/S0140-6736(20)31189-2.

7   Tartof, Sara Y., Lei Qian, Vennis Hong, Rong Wei, Ron F. Nadjafi, Heidi Fischer,
    Zhuoxin Li, et al. "Obesity and Mortality Among Patients Diagnosed With
    COVID-19: Results from an Integrated Health Care Organization." *Annals of
    Internal Medicine* 173, no. 10 (November 17, 2020):773-781. https://www.
    acpjournals.org/doi/full/10.7326/M20-3742.

8   Kyle, Theodore K., Emily J. Dhurandhar, and David B. Allison. "Regarding
    Obesity as a Disease: Evolving Policies and Their Implications." *Endocrinology and
    Metabolism Clinics of North America* 45, no. 3 (September 2016): 511–520. https://
    doi.org/10.1016/j.ecl.2016.04.004.

9   CDC. "Adult Obesity Facts." Last modified February 11, 2021. https://www.cdc.
    gov/obesity/data/adult.html.

10 Kyle, Theodore K., Emily J. Dhurandhar, and David B. Allison. "Regarding Obesity
    as a Disease: Evolving Policies and Their Implications." *National Library of Medicine*
    43, no. 3, (September 2016): 511⊠20. 10.1016/j.ecl.2016.04.004.

11   Kyle, Dhurandhar, and Allison, "Regarding Obesity."

12   Malhotra, Aseem. "COVID-19 and the Elephant in the Room." European Scientist.
      April 16, 2020. https://www.europeanscientist.com/en/article-of-the-week/covid-
      19-and-the-elephant-in-the-room/.

13   Dorsett, Tony. *Running Tough: Memoirs of a Football Maverick.* New York, NY:
      Doubleday, 1989.

14   Lawler, Moira. "8 Ways Weight Loss Can Help Control Diabetes." Everyday
      Health. Last modified November 10. 2020, https://www.everydayhealth.com/hs/
      diabetes-guide-managing-blood-sugar/how-losing-weight-helps/.

15   Volek, Jeff S. and Stephen D. Phinney. *The Art and Science of Low Carbohydrate
      Living: An Expert Guide to Making the Life-Saving Benefits of Carbohydrate Restriction
      Sustainable and Enjoyable.* Beyond Obesity LLC, 2011.

16   Brueck, Hilary. "The Keto Diet Fascinated Americans Most in 2018. Here Are
      the Top 10 Diet Trends of the Year, According to Google." *Business Insider,*
      December 13, 2018. https://www.businessinsider.com/most-popular-diets-keto-
      fodmap-2018-12.

17   Lee, Bruce Y. "Here Are the Top 10 Most Googled Health Questions Of 2019."
      Forbes, December 22, 2019. https://www.forbes.com/sites/brucelee/2019/12/22/
      here-are-the-top-10-most-googled-health-questions-of-2019/?sh=688843a56e77.

18   WebMD. "Ketosis." Last modified May 15, 2020. https://www.webmd.com/
      diabetes/type-1-diabetes-guide/what-is-ketosis#1. Accessed February 26, 2021.

19   Phinney, Stephen and the Virta Team. "What Happens to Triglyceride Levels
      on a Ketogenic Diet?" Virta Health. Accessed February 26, 2021. https://www.
      virtahealth.com/faq/triglycerides-ketogenic-diet.

20   Low Carb USA. "Clinical Guidelines for Therapeutic Carbohydrate Restriction."
      Last modified March 1, 2020. https://www.lowcarbusa.org/wp-content/
      uploads/2020/03/Clinical-Guidelines-General-Intervention-v1.3.7.pdf. Accessed
      February 26, 2021.

21   Volek and Phinney, *The Art and Science of Low Carbohydrate Living.*

22   Critser, Greg. "Legacy of a Fat Man." *Guardian,* September 19, 2003. https://www.
      theguardian.com/theguardian/2003/sep/20/weekend7.weekend1.

23   Volek and Phinney, *The Art and Science of Low Carbohydrate Living.*

24   Volek and Phinney.

25   Volek and Phinney.

26   US Department of Agriculture. "Archived: Food Guide Pyramid." Last modified
      March 20, 2014. https://www.fns.usda.gov/FGP. Accessed February 24, 2021.

27   Teicholz, Nina. *The Big Fat Surprise: Why Butter, Meat and Cheese Belong in a
      Healthy Diet.* New York, NY: Simon & Schuster, 2014.

28   Atkins, Robert. *Dr. Atkins' Diet Revolution: The High Calorie Way to Stay Thin
      Forever.* New York, NY: David McKay, 1972.

29   Atkins. "Atkins' History." Accessed February 26, 2021. https://www.atkins.com/our-story/atkins-diet-history.

30   Fung, Jason. *The Obesity Code: Unlocking the Secrets of Weight Loss.* Vancouver, CA: Greystone Books, 2016.

31   Wartenberg, Lisa. "What is Fat Adaptation?" Healthline. March 5, 2020. https://www.healthline.com/nutrition/fat-adapted.

32   Ghoshal, Malini. "What You Need to Know About Set Point Theory." Healthline. March 19, 2020. https://www.healthline.com/health/set-point-theory.

33   Harvard T.H. Chan School of Public Health. "Carbohydrates and Blood Sugar." Accessed February 24, 2021. https://www.hsph.harvard.edu/nutritionsource/carbohydrates/carbohydrates-and-blood-sugar/.

34   Westman, Eric C. "Is Dietary Carbohydrate Essential for Human Nutrition?" *The American Journal of Clinical Nutrition* 74, no. 5 (May 1, 2002): 951–953. https://doi.org/10.1093/ajcn/75.5.951a.

35   Westman, "Is Dietary Carbohydrate Essential."

36   WebMD. "High Blood Sugar, Diabetes, and Your Body." Last modified December 6, 2020. https://www.webmd.com/diabetes/how-sugar-affects-diabetes/. Accessed February 24, 2021.

37   Villines, Zawn. "How Insulin and Glucagon Regulate Blood Sugar." Medical News Today. March 27, 2019. https://www.medicalnewstoday.com/articles/316427.

38   Cedars Sinai. "Metabolic Syndrome." Accessed February 26, 2021. https://www.cedars-sinai.org/health-library/diseases-and-conditions/m/metabolic-syndrome.html.

39   Spritzler, Franziska. "9 Proven Ways to Fix the Hormones That Control Your Weight." Healthline. March 7, 2016. https://www.healthline.com/nutrition/9-fixes-for-weight-hormones.

40   Legro, Richard S. and Andrea Dunaif. "Menstrual Disorders in Insulin-Resistant States." *Diabetes Spectrum* 10, no. 2 (1997): 185–190. http://journal.diabetes.org/diabetesspectrum/97v10n3/.

41   Fletcher, Jenna. "How Can Diabetes Cause Joint Pain?" Medical News Today. August 29, 2019. https://www.medicalnewstoday.com/articles/326191.

42   American Liver Foundation. "Nonalcoholic Fatty Liver Disease (NAFLD)." Accessed February 26, 2021. https://liverfoundation.org/for-patients/about-the-liver/diseases-of-the-liver/non-alcoholic-fatty-liver-disease/#facts-at-a-glance.

43   Renkl, Margaret. "How Much Do Genes Determine Your Body Type?" Active. Accessed February 24, 2021. https://www.active.com/weight-loss/articles/how-much-do-genes-determine-your-body-type.

44   Tern Fit. "How Accurate Is Your BMI?" Medium. August 14, 2018. https://medium.com/@ternfitteam/how-accurate-is-your-bmi-cdacd0a22e06.

45   Hall, D. M. B. and T. J. Cole. "What Use Is the BMI?" *Archives of Disease in Childhood* 91, no. 4 (March 21, 2006): 283–86. http://dx.doi.org/10.1136/adc.2005.077339.

46   Lawler, "8 Ways Weight Loss Can Help Control Diabetes."

47   Ogunwole, S. Michelle, Cloea A. Zera, and Fatima Cody Stanford. "Obesity Management in Women of Reproductive Age." *JAMA* 325, no. 5 (January 7, 2021): 433–34. https://doi.org/10.1001/jama.2020.21096.

48   Cherney, Kristeen. "A Complete List of Diabetes Medications." Healthline. Last modified June 17, 2020. https://www.healthline.com/health/diabetes/medications-list.

49   American Heart Association. "Types of Heart Medication." Accessed February 26, 2021. https://www.heart.org/en/health-topics/heart-attack/treatment-of-a-heart-attack/cardiac-medications.

50   Hall-Flavin, Daniel K. "Can Antidepressants Cause Weight Gain?" Mayo Clinic. November 17, 2018. https://www.mayoclinic.org/diseases-conditions/depression/expert-answers/antidepressants-and-weight-gain/faq-20058127.

51   Trobisch, Jan. "Medications and Weight." Synergy Wellness. March 16, 2017. https://synergywellnesscenter.com/blog/medications-and-weight/.

52   Trobisch, "Medications and Weight."

53   Trobisch, "Medications and Weight."

54   Byrd-Bredbenner, Carol, Gaile Moe, Jacqueline Berning, and Danita Kelley. *Wardlaw's Perspectives in Nutrition.* New York, NY: McGraw-Hill Education, 2012.

55   USDA National Agricultural Library. "DRI Calculator for Healthcare Professionals." Accessed February 24, 2021. https://www.nal.usda.gov/fnic/dri-calculator/.

56   Layman, Donald K., Tracy G. Anthony, Blake B. Rasmussen, Sean H. Adams, Christopher J. Lynch, Grant D. Brinkworth, and Teresa A. Davis. "Defining Meal Requirements for Proteins to Optimize Metabolic Roles of Amino Acids." *The American Journal of Clinical Nutrition* 101, no. 6 (April 29, 2015): 1330S–1338S. https://doi.org/10.3945/ajcn.114.084053.

57   Houston, D. K., Barbara J. Nicklas, Jingzhong Ding, Tamara B. Harris, Frances A. Tylavsky, Anne B. Newman, Jung Sun Lee, et al. "Dietary Protein Intake Is Associated with Lean Mass Change in Older, Community-Dwelling Adults: The Health, Aging, and Body Composition (Health ABC) Study." *The American Journal of Clinical Nutrition* 87, no. 1 (January 1, 2008): 150–1. https://doi.org/10.1093/ajcn/87.1.150.

58   Siri-Tarino PW, Sun Q, Hu FB, Krauss RM. Meta-analysis of prospective cohort studies evaluating the association of saturated fat with cardiovascular disease. Am J Clin Nutr. 2010 Mar;91(3):535-46.

59   Popkin BM, Hawkes C. The sweetening of the global diet, particularly beverages: patterns, trends and policy responses for diabetes prevention. The Lancet Diabetes & Endocrinology. 2016;4(2):174-186. doi:10.1016/S2213-8587(15)00419-2.

60   Barwell, Anna. "Secret Sugars: The 56 Different Names for Sugar." Virta Health. December 3, 2018. https://www.virtahealth.com/blog/names-for-sugar.

61   Harvard Health Publishing. "The Lowdown on Glycemic Index and Glycemic Load." Last modified April 10, 2020. https://www.health.harvard.edu/diseases-and-conditions/the-lowdown-on-glycemic-index-and-glycemic-load.

62   Glycemic Index Foundation. "Gi Science and Latest Emerging Research." Accessed February 25, 2021. https://www.gisymbol.com/gi-science-and-latest-emerging-research/.

63   Majid, Ameneh, Moira A. Taylor, Alireza Delavari, Reza Malekzadeh, Ian A. Macdonald, Hamid R. Farshchi. "Effects on Weight Loss in Adults of Replacing Diet Beverages with Water during a Hypoenergetic Diet: A Randomized, 24-Week Clinical Trial." *The American Journal of Clinical Nutrition* 102, no. 6 (November 4, 2015): 1305–12. 10.3945/ajcn.115.109397.

64   Sylvetsky, Allison C. and Kristina I. Rother. "Nonnutritive Sweeteners in Weight Management and Chronic Disease." *Obesity* 26, no. 4 (March 23, 2018): 635–40. https://doi.org/10.1002/oby.22139.

65   Yang, Qing. "Gain Weight by 'Going Diet?' Artificial Sweeteners and the Neurobiology of Sugar Cravings." *Yale Journal of Biology and Medicine* 83, no. 2 (June 2010): 101–108. https://www.ncbi.nlm.nih.gov/pmc/articles/PMC2892765/.

66   West, Helen. "How Artificial Sweeteners Affect Blood Sugar and Insulin." Healthline. June 3, 2017. https://www.healthline.com/nutrition/artificial-sweeteners-blood-sugar-insulin.

67   Westman, Eric C., Richard D. Feinman, John C. Mavropoulos, Mary C. Vernon, Jeff S. Volek, James A. Wortman, William S. Yancy, Stephen D. Phinney. "Low-Carbohydrate Nutrition and Metabolism." *American Journal of Clinical Nutrition* 86, no. 2 (August 1, 2007): 276–84. https://doi.org/10.1093/ajcn/86.2.276.

68   Boyles, Salynn. "Obesity Linked to Lower Vitamin D Levels." WebMD. December 17, 2010. https://www.webmd.com/vitamins-and-supplements/news/20101217/obesity-linked-lower-vitamin-d-levels.

69   Stroebel, Charles. *QR: The Quieting Reflex*. New York, NY: Berkley, 1985.

70   Cuncic, Arlin. "How to Practice Progressive Muscle Relaxation." Verywell Mind. Last modified August 3, 2020. https://www.verywellmind.com/how-do-i-practice-progressive-muscle-relaxation-3024400.

71   "Team Shojin. Gokan no Ge." Accessed February 25, 2021. http://teamshojin.jp/the-wisdom-of-shojin-cooking-2/gokan-no-ge.html.

72   Kulkarni, Kshma. Marie Schow, and Jay H. Shubrook. "Shift Workers at Risk for Metabolic Syndrome." *Journal of the American Osteopathic Association* 120, no. 2 (February 1, 2020): 107–17. https://doi.org/10.7556/jaoa.2020.020.

73   Mullington, Janet M., Norah S. Simpson, Hans K. Meier-Ewert, and Monika Haack. "Sleep Loss and Inflammation." *Best Practice & Research: Clinical Endocrinology & Metabolism* 24, no. 5 (October 2010): 775–84. 10.1016/j.beem.2010.08.014.

74   Winter, Bud L. *Relax and Win: Championship Performance in Whatever You Do.* Oak Tree, 1981.

75   Connolly, Josephine, Theresa Romano, and Marisa Patruno. "Effects of Dieting and Exercise on Resting Metabolic Rate and Implications for Weight Management." *Family Practice* 16, no. 2 (April 1999): 196⊠201. https://doi.org/10.1093/fampra/16.2.196.

76   Mawer, Rudy. "Ghrelin: The 'Hunger Hormone' Explained." Healthline. Last modified June 24, 2016. https://www.healthline.com/nutrition/ghrelin.

77   Gunnars, Kris. "How Intermittent Fasting Can Help You Lose Weight." Healthline. Last modified September 25, 2020. https://www.healthline.com/nutrition/intermittent-fasting-and-weight-loss.

78   Fung, *The Obesity Code.*

79   Snyder, Kevin C. "What 'Success' Really Looks Like." *Dr. Kevin C. Snyder* (blog). Accessed February 25, 2021, https://www.kevincsnyder.com/what-success-really-looks-like/.

80   Eenfeldt, Andreas. "The Keto Flu, Other Keto Side Effects, and How to Cure Them." Diet Doctor. Last modified January 7, 2021. https://www.dietdoctor.com/low-carb/keto/flu-side-effects.

81   Eenfeldt, "The Keto Flu."

82   Rada, P., N.M. Avena, and B.G. Hoebel. "Daily Bingeing on Sugar Repeatedly Releases Dopamine in the Accumbens Shell." *Neuroscience* 134, no. 3 (April 16, 2005): 737–44. https://doi.org/10.1016/j.neuroscience.2005.04.043.

83   Volek, Jeff S., Stephen D. Phinney, Cassandra E. Forsythe, Erin E. Quann, Richard J. Wood, Michael J. Puglisi, William J. Kraemer, Doug M. Bibus, Maria Luz Fernandez, and Richard D. Feinman. "Carbohydrate Restriction has a More Favorable Impact on the Metabolic Syndrome than a Low Fat Diet." *Lipids* 44, no.4 (December 12, 2008): 297–309. https://doi.org/10.1007/s11745-008-3274-2.

84   Medline Plus. "Congenital Leptin Deficiency." Accessed February 25, 2021. https://medlineplus.gov/genetics/condition/congenital-leptin-deficiency/.

85   PlushCare. "Consult Live Doctors Online." Accessed February 26, 2021. https://plushcare.com/.

86   Volek, Jeff and Stephen Phinney. "The Sad Saga of Saturated Fat." Virta Health. May 5, 2017. https://www.virtahealth.com/blog/the-sad-saga-of-saturated-fat.

87   Piedmont Healthcare. "Good vs. Bad Cholesterol." Accessed February 25, 2021. https://www.piedmont.org/living-better/good-vs-bad-cholesterol.

88   Piedmont Healthcare, "Good vs. Bad Cholesterol."

89   Sacks, Frank M. and Hannia Campos. "Low-Density Lipoprotein Size and Cardiovascular Disease: A Reappraisal." *The Journal of Clinical Endocrinology & Metabolism* 88, no. 10 (October 1, 2003): 4525–32. https://doi.org/10.1210/jc.2003-030636.

90 Moore, Jimmy and Eric C. Westman. *Cholesterol Clarity: What the HDL is Wrong with my Numbers?* Las Vegas, NV: Victory Belt Publishing, 2013.

91 Hallberg, Sarah J., Amy L. McKenzie, Paul T. Williams, Nasir H. Bhanpuri, Anne L. Peters, Wayne W. Campbell, Tamara L. Hazbun, et al. "Effectiveness and Safety of a Novel Care Model for the Management of Type 2 Diabetes at Year 1: An Open Label, Non-Randomized Controlled Study." *Diabetes Therapy* 9 (February 7, 2018): 583–612. https://doi.org/10.1007/s13300-018-0373-9.

92 Hallberg, "Effectiveness and Safety."

93 Johnston, Anita. *Eating in the Light of the Moon: How Women Can Transform Their Relationship with Food Through Myths, Metaphors, and Storytelling.* Nashville, TN: Gürze Books, 2000.

94 Johnson, Anita. "Dr. Anita Johnston – Eating in the Light of the Moon." n.d. https://dranitajohnston.com/.

95 Kabat-Zinn, Jon. *Wherever You Go, There You Are: Mindfulness Meditation in Everyday Life.* New York, NY: Hachette, 2005.

96 Meyers, Jonathan. "Exercise and Cardiovascular Health." *Circulation* 107, no. 1 (January 7, 2003): e2–e3. https://www.ahajournals.org/doi/10.1161/01.CIR.0000048890.59383.8D.

97 Kritz-Silverstein, Donna, Elizabeth Barrett-Connor, and Catherine Corbeau. "Cross-Sectional and Prospective Study of Exercise and Depressed Mood in the Elderly: The Rancho Bernardo Study." *American Journal of Epidemiology* 153, no. 6 (March 15, 2001): 596–603. https://doi.org/10.1093/aje/153.6.596.

98 Forman, D. "Exercise: 15 Minutes a Day Ups Lifespan by 3 Years." Harvard Health Publishing. December 2013. https://www.health.harvard.edu/heart-health/exercise-15-minutes-a-day-ups-lifespan-by-3-years.

99 Klissouras, V. "Heritability of Adaptive Variation." *Journal of Applied Physiology* 31, no. 3 (September 1971): 338–44. https://doi.org/10.1152/jappl.1971.31.3.338.

100 Woo, R., J S Garrow, and F X Pi-Sunyer. "Voluntary Food Intake during Prolonged Exercise in Obese Women." *American Journal of Clinical Nutrition* 36, no. 3 (September 1982): 478–84. https://doi.org/10.1093/ajcn/36.3.478.

101 Phinney, Stephen D., Betty M. LaGrange, Maureen O'Connell, and Elliot Danforth Jr. "Effects of Aerobic Exercise on Energy Expenditure and Nitrogen Balance during Very Low Calorie Dieting." *Metabolism* 37, no. 8 (August 1, 1988): 758–65. https://doi.org/10.1016/0026-0495(88)90011-X.

102 Janney, Carol A. and John M. Jakicic. "The Influence of Exercise and BMI on Injuries and Illnesses in Overweight and Obese Individuals: A Randomized Control Trial." *International Journal of Behavioral Nutrition and Physical Activity* 7, no. 1 (January 6, 2010). https://doi.org/10.1186/1479-5868-7-1.

103 Science Daily. "Exercise Is More Critical Than Diet to Maintain Weight Loss." March 29, 2019. https://www.sciencedaily.com/releases/2019/03/190329130227.htm.

104 Bays, HE, W. McCarthy, S. Christensen, J. Seger, S. Wells, J. Long, and N.N. Shah. "Obesity Algorithm Slides." Obesity Medicine Association. 2019. https://obesitymedicine.org/obesity-algorithm-powerpoint/.

105 US Department of Health and Human Services, Food and Drug Administration, and Center for Drug Evaluation and Research (CDER). "Guidance for Industry Developing Products for Weight Management." FDA.gov. February 2007. https://www.fda.gov/media/71252/download.

106 National Institute of Diabetes and Digestive and Kidney Diseases. "Prescription Medications to Treat Overweight and Obesity." July 2016. https://www.niddk.nih.gov/health-information/weight-management/prescription-medications-treat-overweight-obesity/.

107 Stanford, Fatima Cody, Nasreen Alfaris, Gricelda Gomez, Elizabeth T. Ricks, Alpana P. Shukla, Kathleen E. Corey, Janey S. Pratt, Alfons Pomp, Francesco Rubino, and Louis J. Aronne. "The Utility of Weight Loss Medications after Bariatric Surgery for Weight Regain or Inadequate Weight Loss: A Multi-Center Study." *Surgery for Obesity and Related Diseases* 13, no. 3 (October 27, 2016): 491–500. https://doi.org/10.1016/j.soard.2016.10.018.

108 National Institute of Diabetes and Digestive and Kidney Diseases. "Prescription Medications."

109 Hendricks, Ed J. "Off-Label Drugs for Weight Management." *Diabetes, Metabolic Syndrome and Obesity: Targets and Therapy* 10, (June 10, 2017): 223–34. https://doi.org/10.2147/DMSO.S95299.

110 Lee, P. C., S. Ganguly, and S.-Y. Goh. "Weight Loss Associated with Sodium-Glucose Cotransporter-2 Inhibition: A Review of Evidence and Underlying Mechanisms." *Obesity Reviews* 19, no. 12 (September 25, 2018): 1630–41. https://doi.org/10.1111/obr.12755.

111 Diaz-Ramos, Alexis, Wesley Eilbert, and Diego Marquez. "Euglycemic Diabetic Ketoacidosis Associated with Sodium-Glucose Cotransporter-2 Inhibitor Use: A Case Report and Review of the Literature." *International Journal of Emergency Medicine* 12, no. 27 (September 5, 2019). https://doi.org/10.1186/s12245-019-0240-0.

112 Harvard Health Publishing. "Thyroid Hormone: Slim Fast, but Will It Last?" September 2007. https://www.health.harvard.edu/newsletter_article/thyroid_hormone_slim_fast_but_will_it_last/.

113 Northwestern Medicine. "I'm Gaining Weight, Is It My Thyroid?" Accessed February 26, 2021. https://www.nm.org/healthbeat/healthy-tips/im-gaining-weight-is-it-my-thyroid.

114 American Society for Metabolic and Bariatric Surgery (ASMBS). "Benefits of Weight Loss Surgery." Last modified September 2020. https://asmbs.org/patients/benefits-of-weight-loss-surgery.

115 ASMBS. "Benefits of Weight Loss Surgery."

116 Herman, Katya M., Tamara E. Carver, Nicolas V. Christou, and Ross E. Andersen. "Keeping the Weight Off: Physical Activity, Sitting Time, and Weight Loss

Maintenance in Bariatric Surgery Patients 2 to 16 Years Postsurgery." *Obesity Surgery* 24, no. 7 (February 28, 2014): 1064–72. https://doi.org/10.1007/s11695-014-1212-3.

117 ASMBS. "Benefits of Weight Loss Surgery."

118 Metabolic and Bariatric Surgery Accreditation and Quality Improvement (MBSAQIP). "Optimal Resources for Metabolic and Bariatric Surgery, 2019 Standards." American College of Surgeons. 2019. https://www.facs.org/-/media/files/quality-programs/bariatric/2019_mbsaqip_standards_manual.ashx.

119 Lim, Robert B. "Bariatric Procedures for the Management of Severe Obesity: Descriptions." UpToDate.com. Last modified November 18, 2020. https://www.uptodate.com/contents/bariatric-procedures-for-the-management-of-severe-obesity-descriptions.

120 WebMD. "Choosing a Type of Weight Loss Surgery." Nourish. Accessed February 26, 2021. https://www.webmd.com/diet/obesity/weight-loss-surgery-making-the-choice#1.

121 Cohen, Pieter A. "Hazards of Hindsight—Monitoring the Safety of Nutritional Supplements." *The New England Journal of Medicine* 370, (April 3, 2014): 1277-1280. https://doi.org/10.1056/NEJMp1315559.

122 Interlandi, Jeneen. "Some Weight Loss Pills Still Contain Banned Substances." Consumer Reports. August 17, 2016. https://www.consumerreports.org/vitamins-supplements/weight-loss-pills-stil-contain-banned-ingredients/.

123 Scheen, André J. "Sibutramine on Cardiovascular Outcome." *Diabetes Care* 34, no. 2 (May 2011): S114–S119. https://doi.org/10.2337/dc11-s205.

124 Halperin, Florencia. "Weight-Loss Drug Belviq Recalled." Harvard Health Publishing. April 9, 2020. https://www.health.harvard.edu/blog/weight-loss-drug-belviq-recalled-2020040919439.

125 Bays HE, "Obesity Algorithm Slides."

126 Han, Yong, Lei Zhang, Xiang-Qun Liu, Zhi-Jun Zhao, and Lu-Xian Lv. "Effect of Glucomannan on Functional Constipation in Children: A Systematic Review and Meta-Analysis of Randomised Controlled Trials." *Asia Pacific Journal of Clinical Nutrition* 26, no. 3 (May 2017): 471–477. 10.6133/apjcn.032016.03.

127 Usp.org. "US Pharmacopeia (USP)." 2019. https://www.usp.org/.

128 TRC Health. "Natural Medicines." Accessed February 26, 2021. https://info.therapeuticresearch.com/natural-medicines-organic-social/.

129 Hairston, Kristen G., Mara Z. Vitolins, Jill M. Norris, Andrea M. Anderson, Anthony J. Hanley, and Lynne E. Wagenknecht. "Lifestyle Factors and 5-Year Abdominal Fat Accumulation in a Minority Cohort: The IRAS Family Study." *Obesity* 20, no. 2 (September 6, 2012): 421–427. https://doi.org/10.1038/oby.2011.171.

130 Van De Walle, Gavin. "Do Exogenous Ketone Supplements Work for Weight Loss?" Healthline. October 23, 2018. https://www.healthline.com/nutrition/exogenous-ketones.

131 Yang, Chung S., Gang Chen, and Qing Wu. "Recent Scientific Studies of a Traditional Chinese Medicine, Tea, on Prevention of Chronic Diseases." *Journal of Traditional and Complementary Medicine* 4, no. 1 (January–March 2014): 17–23. https://doi.org/10.4103/2225-4110.124326.

132 Jurgens, Tannis and Anne Marie Whelan. "Can Green Tea Preparations Help with Weight Loss?" *Canadian Pharmacists Journal* 147, no. 3 (March 31, 2014): 159–160. https://doi.org/10.1177/1715163514528668.

133 Schubert, Matthew M., Christopher Irwin, Rebekah F. Seay, Holly E. Clarke, Deanne Allegro, and Ben Desbrow. "Caffeine, Coffee, and Appetite Control: A Review." *International Journal of Food Sciences and Nutrition* 68, no. 8 (April 27, 2017): 901–12. https://doi.org/10.1080/09637486.2017.1320537.

134 Chen, Kim, John Pullman, Timothy Bailey, Ken Fujioka, Mark Tager, and Martin Brown. "Effectiveness of the LOVIDIA Way, a Combination of Lovidia Hunger Control Formula Taken Daily with Intermittent Calorie Restriction for Weight Management and Metabolic Health." https://36hg0x2qkb4e2n3u3asvcokq-wpengine.netdna-ssl.com/wp-content/uploads/2018/12/lovidia-way-study-results.pdf.

135 Robertson, Ruairi. "Omega-3-6-9 Fatty Acids: A Complete Overview." Healthline. Last modified October 22, 2020. https://www.healthline.com/nutrition/omega-3-6-9-overview.

136 Buettner, Dan. "Hara Hachi Bu: Enjoy Food and Lose Weight with This Simple Japanese Phrase." Blue Zones. Last modified December 2018. https://www.bluezones.com/2017/12/hara-hachi-bu-enjoy-food-and-lose-weight-with-this-simple-phrase/.

137 Moorhouse, Drusilla. "This Fitness Trend Is a Hit with People Who Love Exercise and the Environment." BuzzFeed News. January 13, 2019. https://www.buzzfeednews.com/article/drumoorhouse/what-is-plogging-environment-swedish-fitness-trend.

Made in the USA
Monee, IL
18 October 2021